SIRTFOOD

Sirtfood Diet: 51 Simple and Tasty

Recipes That Will Activate Your

"Skinny Gene" That Burns Fat Fast

Jamie Smipool

Contents

INTRODUCTION

Sirtfood Diet was created by two celebrity nutritionists working with a private gym in the UK.

They market the diet as a radical modern lifestyle and wellness program that works by flipping the "skinny switch" on.

This diet is focused on sirtuin research (SIRTs), a community of seven proteins contained in the body that has been shown to control a number of functions, including metabolism, inflammation, and lifespan;

Some compounds of natural plants increase the body's protein, and the foods it contains are referred to as 'sirt foods.'

The Sirtfood Diet's creators are Aidan Goggins and Glen Matte, both professional nutritionists who succeeded in harnessing the influence of 'Sirtfood' research to build a groundbreaking diet.

The science behind the diet is all about these Sirtfoods, a group of newly discovered daily plant foods high in a chemical compound known as sirtuin activators.

These sirtuin activators are a type of protein that flips on the body pathways of the so-called 'skinny gene.'

These slim pathways are the same ones that are stimulated more frequently through fasting and exercise, which help the body lose weight, raise muscle mass, and boosts your fitness. Countries where people are now consuming a substantial amount of Sirtfoods as part of their conventional diet, like Japan and Italy, are also consistently ranked among the world's healthiest.

Is Sirtfoods the New Superfoods?

Now that we've all heard of alkaline diet, paleo, raw food, vegan or gluten-free, but the latest trend to reach the health and fitness market is sirtfood, which is hailed as a modern, somewhat 'social' superfood. Gone are days of restrictive diet plans to deter you from having dinner with friends or going to a nightclub, party or restaurant. Instead, the sirtfood diet is red wine, coffee and chocolate friendly, all rich in sirtuin activators believed to improve the immune system and help you lose weight.

The Sirtfood diet, which was first introduced in 2016, remains a popular topic and entails adherents following a diet abundant in 'sirt foods.' Such unique foods function by stimulating different proteins in the body called sirtuins, according to the diet's creators. Sirtuins are thought to prevent the body's cells from dying while under heat and are thought to control inflammation, metabolism, and aging. Sirtuins are believed to affect the body 's capacity to lose fat and improve metabolism, resulting in a weight reduction of seven pounds a week while retaining the muscle. However, some researchers say this is unlikely to be simply a fat reduction but may represent improvements in skeletal muscle and liver glycogen stocks instead.

The diet is split into two phases; the initial period lasts one week and includes a three-day reduction in calories to 1000 kcal, intake in three sirtfood green juices and one meal rich in sirt foods. The juices contain spinach, celery, rocket, parsley, lemon and green tea. Meals contain turkey escalope with buckwheat noodles, basil, capers and parsley, chicken and kale curry, and prawn stir-fry. Energy intakes from days four to seven are increased to 1500kcal, consisting of two sirtfood green juices and two sirtfood-rich meals a day.

Even though the diet promotes healthy foods, it is restrictive, especially during the initial stages, in both your food choices and daily calories. It also includes consuming water, with the recommended quantities meeting the existing average requirements during step one.

The second period is regarded as the 14-day maintenance process, where there is a slow weight loss. The writers think it's a practical and safe way to lose weight. Focusing on weight reduction, though, is not what the diet is about – it's supposed to be about consuming the best food that nature has to bring. They suggest three healthy sirtfood-rich meals a day together with one sirtfood-green juice in the long term.

PHASE 1 AND PHASE 2 OF THE SIRTFOOD DIET

The Sirtfood Diet has two phases that last three weeks altogether. You can then continue to "sirtify" your diet by including as many sirt foods as possible into your meals. The basic recipes for these two phases can be found in the book The Sirtfood Diet, which was published by makers of the diet. There are many sirt foods in the meals, but other food items are in addition to the "top 20 sirt foods."

Most sirtfoods and ingredients are easy to find. Three of the signature ingredients required for these two phases — matcha green tea powder, lovage, and buckwheat — may, however, be costly or hard to find.

A large part of the diet is its green juice, which you'll have to make between one and three times a day. A juicer (a blender won't work) and a kitchen scale will be needed, as the ingredients are listed by weight. The recipe is below:

- ✓ Sirtfood Green Juice
- ✓ 75 grams (2.5 oz) kale
- ✓ 30 grams (1 oz) arugula (rocket)

- ✓ five grams parsley
- ✓ two celery sticks
- ✓ one cm (0.5 in) ginger
- ✓ ½ of a green apple
- ✓ ½ of a lemon
- ✓ ½ of a teaspoon matcha green tea

juice all ingredients except green tea powder and lemon, and pour into a glass. Squeeze the lemon by hand, then mix the lemon juice and green tea powder into the juice.

Phase One

The first phase lasts for seven days, with calorie restriction and lots of green juice involved. It's meant to boost your weight loss and claim to help you lose 7 pounds (3.2 kg) in seven days.

Intake of calories during the first three days of phase one is limited to 1,000 calories. You drink three green drinks, plus one dish, every day. You will select from recipes in the book every day, many of which include sirtfood as a big part of the meal.

E.g., miso-glazed tofu, the omelet sirtfood, or the buckwheat stir-fry shrimp. On days 4-7 of Phase One, calorie consumption is raised to 1,500. This involves two green juices a day and two more sirt-rich meals that can be picked from the book.

Phase Two

Phase two takes two weeks to complete. You should continue to loose weight steadily during this "maintenance" phase.

This phase has no specific calorie limit. Instead, you eat three sirt-fed meals and one green juice a day. The meals are again selected from the recipes found in the book.

After the Diet

Those two stages can be replicated as much as you want for more weight reduction. However, after completing those phases, you are encouraged to continue "sirtifying" your diet by regularly incorporating sirt foods into your meals.

LIST OF SIRTFOODS

✓ Kale

- ✓ Red wine
- ✓ Strawberries
- ✓ Onions
- ✓ Soy
- ✓ Parsley
- ✓ Extra virgin olive oil
- ✓ Dark chocolate (85% cocoa)
- ✓ Matcha green tea
- ✓ Buckwheat
- ✓ Turmeric
- ✓ Walnuts
- ✓ Arugula (rocket)
- ✓ Bird's eye chili
- ✓ Lovage
- ✓ Medjool dates
- ✓ Red chicory
- ✓ Blueberries
- ✓ Capers
- ✓ Coffee

The makers of the diet say that adopting the Sirtfood diet would result in rapid weight loss, thus retaining muscle mass and shielding you from chronic disease.

Once you've finished the program, you 're encouraged to resume your regular diet with sirt products and the popular green juice of the diet.

HOW GOOD IS THE SIRTFOOD

There's no denying that sirtfoods benefit you. They are frequently high in nutrients and complete healthy plant compounds.

Moreover, research studies have actually associated many of the foods recommended on the Sirtfood Diet with health advantages.

For example, consuming moderate amounts of dark chocolate with high cocoa content might decrease the danger of cardiovascular disease and assistance fight inflammation.

Consuming green tea might decrease the risk of stroke and diabetes and help lower high blood pressure.

And turmeric has anti-inflammatory properties that have advantageous impacts on the body in general and may even secure against chronic, inflammation-related illness).

The bulk of sirtfoods have actually demonstrated health benefits in people.

Nevertheless, proof of the health advantages of increasing sirtuin protein levels is preliminary. Research in animals and cell lines has revealed exciting results.

For instance, researchers have found that increased levels of certain sirtuin proteins cause longer lifespan in yeast, mice, and worms.

And throughout fasting or calorie limitation, sirtuin proteins inform the body to burn more fat for energy and improve insulin level of sensitivity. One study in mice discovered that increased sirtuin levels resulted in weight loss.

Some evidence recommends that sirtuins may likewise play a role in minimizing swelling, hindering the advancement of growths, and slowing the development of cardiovascular disease and Alzheimer's.

While research studies in mice and human cell lines have revealed favorable results, there have been no human studies examining the effects of increasing sirtuin levels.

Whether increasing sirtuin protein levels in the body will lead to longer life-span or a lower danger of cancer in humans is unknown.

Research study is currently underway to develop substances efficient at increasing sirtuin levels in the body. By doing this, human research studies can begin to take a look at the effects of sirtuins on human health

Until then, it's not possible to identify the results of increased sirtuin levels.

Sirtfoods are generally healthy foods. Extremely little is understood about how these foods affect sirtuin levels and human health.

Is It Effective?

The Sirtfood Diet's authors make bold statements that the diet will overburden weight loss, turn on the "lene gene," and avoid illness.

There is little evidence to support the problem.

Far from it, there is no persuasive evidence that Sirtfood Diet has a more positive weight loss effect than any other limited calorie diet.

And although numerous of these foods have healthful homes, there have not been any long-lasting human research studies to determine whether eating a diet rich in sirtfoods has any concrete health benefits.

Nonetheless, this sirtfood diet plan book reports the outcomes of a pilot study conducted by the authors and involving 39 individuals from their gym. Nevertheless, the results of this study appear not to have been published anywhere else.

For one week, the individuals followed the diet and worked out daily. At the end of the week, participants lost approximately 7 pounds (3.2 kg) and kept or perhaps gained muscle mass.

Yet these outcomes are hardly surprising. Restricting your calorie intake to 1,000 calories and working out at the very same time will almost always trigger weight reduction.

Regardless, this type of quick weight-loss is neither lasting nor genuine, and this study did not follow participants after the very first week to see if they got any of the weight back, which is normally the case.

When your body is energy-deprived, it utilizes up its emergency situation energy stores, or glycogen, in addition to burning fat and muscle.

Each particle of glycogen needs 3-- 4 particles of water to be kept. It gets rid of the water when your body is using glycogen. It is called the "weight of the water."

Only about one-third of weight loss comes from fat in the first week of extreme calorie stress, and the other two thirds from water, muscle and glycogen

As your calories increase, the body renovates its glycogen reserves, and the weight recovers instantly.

This type of calorie limitation can likewise cause your body to decrease its metabolic rate, triggering you require even fewer calories per day for energy than before

It is most likely that this diet plan may assist you to lose a couple of pounds in the beginning, but it will likely come back as quickly as the diet plan is over.

As far as avoiding illness, three weeks is probably not long enough to have any measurable long-lasting effect.

On another hand, it might still be a smart thing to add sirt food to your daily diet in the long run. You should still stop your diet in that case, and start doing so now.

This diet may assist you to drop weight since it is low in calories, but the weight is most likely to return when the diet plan ends. The diet plan is too short of having a long-term impact on your health.

Is It Healthy And Sustainable?

Sirtfoods are nearly all healthy options and may even lead to some health benefits due to their anti-inflammatory or antioxidant residential or commercial properties.

Yet consuming simply a handful of particularly healthy foods can not satisfy all of your body's dietary needs.

The Sirtfood Diet is needlessly restrictive and uses no clear, special health benefits over any other kind of diet.

Eating only 1,000 calories is normally not suggested without the supervision of a physician. Even consuming 1,500 calories per day is exceedingly limiting for many individuals.

The diet plan also needs draining to 3 green juices per day. Although juices can be a good source of minerals and vitamins, they are likewise a source of sugar and consist of nearly none of the healthy fiber that whole fruits and veggies do

What's more, sipping on juice throughout the whole day is a bad concept for both your blood sugar and your teeth.

Not to point out, because the diet plan is so minimal in calories and food choice, it is more than most likely lacking in protein, vitamins, and minerals, specifically during the first stage.

Due to the low-calorie levels and limiting food options, this diet plan may be challenging to adhere to for the whole three weeks.

Add that to the high initial expenses of needing to buy a juicer, the book, and specific uncommon and costly components, in addition to the time expenses of preparing specific meals and juices, and this diet plan ends up being unfeasible and unsustainable for many individuals.

The Sirtfood Diet promotes healthy foods but is limiting in calories and food choices. It likewise involves drinking great deals of juice, which isn't a healthy suggestion.

HOW TO MAINTAIN THE HEALTHY WEIGHT GAINED WITH THE SIRT DIET

Combining Exercise With The Sirtfood Diet

With 52% of Americans admitting that they discover it simpler to do their taxes than to comprehend how to consume healthily, it's crucial to introduce a kind of eating that becomes a lifestyle rather than a one-off crash diet. For a few of us, it may not be that tough to drop weight or retain a healthy weight; however, the Sirtfood diet plan can assist those who are struggling. What about integrating the Sirtfood diet plan with a workout, is it a good idea to prevent exercise entirely or present it when you have begun the diet plan?

The SirtDiet Principles

With an estimated 650 million obese adults globally, it's essential to find healthy eating and exercise routines that are achievable, don't deny you of whatever you delight in, and don't require you to work out all week. The Sirtfood diet does just that. The concept is that particular foods will activate the 'skinny gene' pathways, which are typically activated by fasting and exercise. The bright side is that particular food and beverage, consisting of dark chocolate and red wine, consists of chemicals called polyphenols that trigger the genes that imitate the results of exercise and fasting.

Exercise during the first few weeks

During the very first week or two of the diet plan where your calorie intake is minimized, it would be sensible to stop or lower workout while your body adjusts to fewer calories. Understand the body, and don't do exercise if you are exhausted or have less strength than normal. Rather ensure that you stay focused on the principles that use to a healthy lifestyle such as consisting of sufficient everyday levels of fiber, protein and fruit and veggies.

When the diet becomes a lifestyle

When you do exercise, it's important to take in protein, preferably an hour after your workout. Protein repair work muscles after a workout lower pain and can aid healing. There are various types of sauces, including the sirt chili con carne, or the turmeric chicken and the kale salad, which are suitable for after exercise consumptions. If you desire something lighter, you could try the sirt blueberry healthy smoothie and include some protein powder for added advantage. The kind of physical fitness you do will be down to you; however, exercises in the house will permit you to select when to exercise, the types of workouts that fit you and are short and hassle-free.

The Sirtfood diet is a fantastic way to change your eating practices, reduce weight and feel healthier. The preliminary few weeks may challenge you, but it is necessary to examine which foods are best to consume and which scrumptious recipes match you. Be kind to yourself in the first couple of weeks while your body adapts and takes exercise easy if you select to do it at all. If you are already somebody who does extreme or moderate exercise, then it might be that you can continue as typical or manage your physical fitness in accordance with the change in diet. Similar to any diet plan and workout changes, it's

everything about the private and how far you can press
yourself.

SIRTFOOD RECIPES

1. Sirtfood Bites

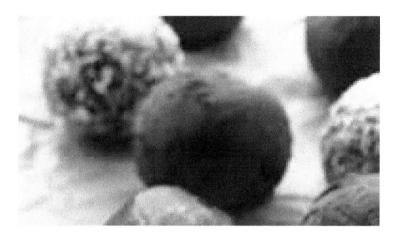

Ingredients:

- ✓ (85% cocoa solids), 1 ounce (30g) dark chocolate, 1/4 cup cocoa nibs or broken into pieces;
- ✓ 1 cup (120g) walnuts
- ✓ pitted, 9 ounces (250g) Medjool dates
- ✓ One tablespoon ground turmeric
- ✓ One tablespoon cocoa powder
- ✓ the scraped seeds of 1 vanilla pod or one teaspoon vanilla extract
- ✓ One tablespoon extra virgin olive oil
- ✓ 1 to 2 tablespoons of water

Instructions:

✓ Place the walnuts and the chocolate in a food processor and then Proceed until you've got a fine powder.

✓ Add all other ingredients other than water and combine until a ball is shaped. Depending on the consistency of the mixture, you may or may not add the water — you don't want that to be too adhesive.

✓ Formake a bite-sized paste with your hands and cool down for at least 1 hour in an airtight jar before consuming them.

✓ You can roll some of the balls to a different finish if you want to in some cocoa or dried cocoa. And can be store in your fridge for up to one week.

2. Sirt Super Salad

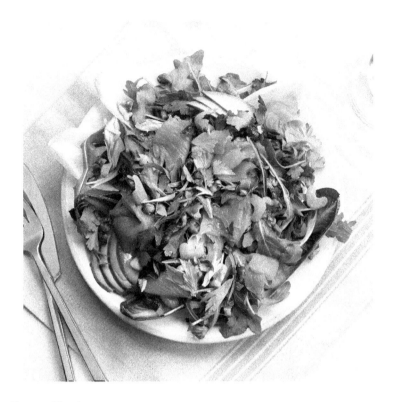

Ingredients:

- ✓ 1 3⁄4 ounces (50g) endive leaves
- ✓ 1 3⁄4 ounces (50g) arugula
- ✓ 3 1⁄2 ounces (100g) smoked salmon slices
- ✓ 1⁄2 cup (50g) celery including leaves, sliced
- ✓ 1⁄2 cup (80g) avocado, peeled, stoned, and sliced
- ✓ 1⁄8 cups (15g) walnuts, chopped
- ✓ 1⁄8 cup (20g) red onion, sliced

- ✓ One tablespoon capers
- ✓ One tablespoon extra virgin olive oil
- ✓ One large Medjool date, pitted and chopped
- ✓ juice of 1/4 lemon
- ✓ 1/4 cup (10g) parsley, chopped

Instructions:

- ✓ In a plate or wide cup, position the salad leaves.
- ✓ Mix all the remainder of the ingredients and pour over the seeds.

3. Miso-Marinated Baked Cod With Stir-Fried Greens And Sesame

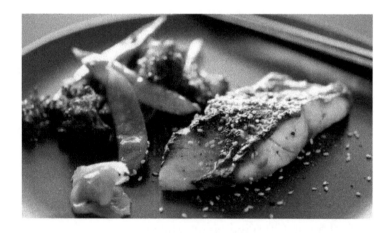

Ingredients:

- ✓ One tablespoon extra virgin olive oil
- ✓ 3 1⁄2 teaspoons (20g) miso
- ✓ One tablespoon mirin
- ✓ 1⁄8 cup (20g) red onion, sliced
- ✓ 1 x 7-ounce (200g) skinless cod fillet
- ✓ Two garlic cloves, finely chopped
- ✓ 3⁄8 cup (40g) celery, sliced
- ✓ One teaspoon finely chopped fresh ginger
- ✓ One Thai chili, finely chopped
- ✓ 3⁄4 cup (50g) kale, roughly chopped
- ✓ 3⁄8 cup (60g) green beans
- ✓ Two tablespoons (5g) parsley, roughly chopped
- ✓ One teaspoon sesame seeds
- ✓ 1⁄4 cup (40g) buckwheat
- ✓ One tablespoon tamari (or soy sauce, if not avoiding gluten)
- ✓ One teaspoon ground turmeric

Instructions:

- ✓ Combine the miso, mirin and one oil tea cubicle. Rub the whole cod and set for 30 minutes to marinate. Oven heated to 220 degrees C (425 degrees F).
- ✓ Bake the cod for 10 minutes.
- ✓ Heat the remaining oil in a large frying pan or wok. Remove the celery, garlic, chili, ginger, green beans, and kale and deep fry for a few minutes. Sprinkle and sprinkle until the kale is soft and baked. To help the cooking process, you might have to put a bit of water into the pot.
- ✓ Cook buckwheat together with turmeric in accordance with the package instructions.
- ✓ Serve the stir-fry with sesame, parsley and tamari seeds and fish. Serve in the stir-fry.

4. Aromatic Chicken Breast With Kale And Red Onions And A Tomato And Chili Salsa

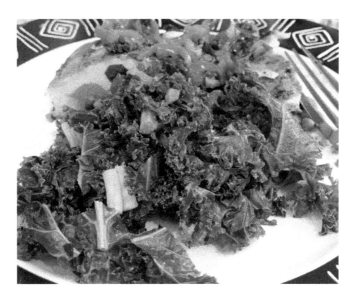

Ingredients:

- ✓ Skinless 1⁄4 pound (120 g), Monotonous chicken breast.
- ✓ Two ground turmeric teaspoons
- ✓ 1/2 lemon juice
- ✓ Extra virgin olive oil one charcoal tablespoon.
- ✓ Three-quarters (50 g) kale, cut off.
- ✓ Red onion cut 1⁄8 cup (20 g)
- ✓ New ginger sliced with one teaspoon
- ✓ 1⁄3 cup of light wheat (50 g);

The Salsa

- ✓ One small (130 g) tomato

- ✓ One Thai chili, deeply sliced.
- ✓ One caper of a teaspoon, fine cut
- ✓ Parsley 2 teaspoons (5 g), fine cut
- ✓ 1/4 lemon of juice

Instructions:

- ✓ Remove the eye from the tomato to make the salsa and pinch it finely, ensuring that the fluid remains as high as possible. Combine chile, capers, lemon juice and parsley. You might mix it all in, but the end product is a little different.
- ✓ Oven to 220 degrees Celsius (425 ° F), in one teaspoon, marinate the chicken breast with a little oil and lemon juice. Leave for five to ten minutes.
- ✓ Then add the marinated chicken and cook on either side for about a minute, until pale golden, transfer to the oven (on a baking tray, if your pan is not ovenproof), 8 to 10 minutes or until cooked. Remove from the oven, cover with tape, and wait until eaten for five minutes.
- ✓ Cook the kale for 5 minutes in a steamer in the meantime, in a little butter, fry the red onions and the ginger and then mix in the fluffy but not browned chalk.

✓ Cook the buckwheat with the remaining turmeric teaspoon according to the package instructions. Eat rice, tomatoes and salsa. Eat together.

5. Asian Shrimp Stir-Fry With Buckwheat Noodles

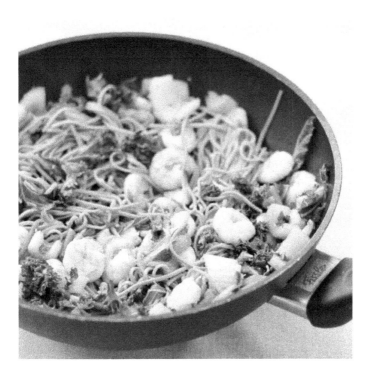

Ingredients:

- ✓ Two teaspoons tamari (you can use soy sauce if you are not avoiding gluten)
- ✓ 1⁄3 pound (150g) shelled raw jumbo shrimp, deveined
- ✓ Two teaspoons extra virgin olive oil
- ✓ Two garlic cloves, finely chopped
- ✓ Three ounces (75g) soba (buckwheat noodles)
- ✓ One teaspoon finely chopped fresh ginger
- ✓ One Thai chili, finely chopped
- ✓ 1⁄2 cup (45g) celery including leaves, trimmed and sliced, with leaves set aside
- ✓ 1⁄8 cup (20g) red onions, sliced
- ✓ 3⁄4 cup (50g) kale, roughly chopped
- ✓ 1⁄2 cup (75g) green beans, chopped
- ✓ 1⁄2 cup (100ml) chicken stock

Instructions:

- ✓ Prepare the pan for high heat, then cook the shrimps for 2 to 3 minutes in 1 tamari tea cubicle and one olive tea cubicle.
- ✓ Switch to a tray of shrimp. Cover the pan with a towel or cloth, and you'll need it again.

- ✓ Cook the noodles 5 to 8 minutes or as indicated on the box in boiling water. Drain and reserve. Drain.
- ✓ Fried in the remaining tamari and oil over half to high heat for 2 to 3 minutes in the garlic, pepper, ginger and red onion, celery (but not the blade). Stir the stock and boil until they are tender, but always crunchy, then simmer for a minute or two.
- ✓ Stir in a pan and put back to boil, then take the shrimp, pasta, and celery leaves from the oven, and drink.

6. Strawberry Buckwheat Tabbouleh

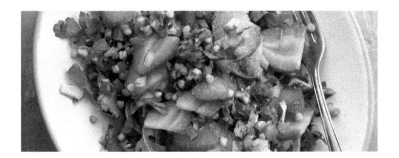

Ingredients:

- ✓ One tablespoon ground turmeric

- ✓ 1/3 cup (50g) buckwheat
- ✓ 1/2 cup (80g) avocado
- ✓ 1/8 cup (20g) red onion
- ✓ 3/8 cup (65g) tomato
- ✓ One tablespoon capers
- ✓ 1/8 cup (25g) Medjool dates, pitted
- ✓ 2/3 cup (100g) strawberries, hulled
- ✓ 3/4 cup (30g) parsley
- ✓ juice of 1/2 lemon
- ✓ One tablespoon extra virgin olive oil
- ✓ 1 ounce (30g) arugula

Instructions:

- ✓ Cook the turmeric with buckwheat according to the directions for the box.
- ✓ Rinse to cool off.
- ✓ Chop the agua finely, peppers, red onions, bananas, capers, and pots, and blend along with the fresh buckwheat.
- ✓ Dice the strawberries and combine the oils with the lemon juice softly in the salad. Serve on arugula bed. MAKES:1 PREP TIME: 10 mins COOK TIME: 3 mins TOTAL TIME: 13 mins

7. Sirtfood Green Juice

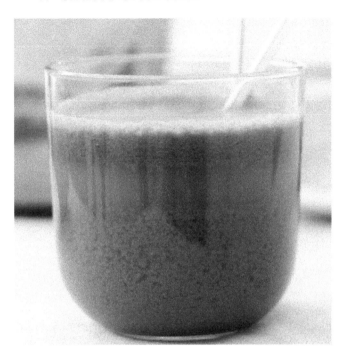

Ingredients:

- ✓ a large handful (1 ounce or 30g) arugula
- ✓ Two large handfuls (about 2 1⁄2 ounces or 75g) kale
- ✓ 2 to 3 large celery stalks (5 1⁄2 ounces or 150g), including leaves
- ✓ a very small handful (about 1⁄4 ounce or 5g) flat-leaf parsley
- ✓ 1/2- to 1-inch (1 to 2.5 cm) piece of fresh ginger
- ✓ 1/2 medium green apple

- ✓ 1/2 level teaspoon matcha powder
- ✓ juice of 1/2 lemon

Instructions:

- ✓ Mix the greens together and then sauté the greens. We discovered that the efficiency of juicers could vary greatly from leafy food to rejuicate the rest of the food, and before moving to other ingredients. The goal is to get approximately 2 or 1/4 cup of green juice or around two fluid ounces.
- ✓ Celery juice, apple, ginger juice
- ✓ You can peel and place the citrus fruit also, but it is much easier just to squeeze the citrus fruits by hand into the juice. By this point, you should have a limit of about 1 cup (250 ml) of water.
- ✓ You just add the matcha if the juice is cooked and ready to drink. Into a glass, add a small amount of the juice and mix with a blaze or teaspoon vigorously.
- ✓ Add the rest of the juice when the matcha is dissolved. Give it a quick swirl, and then drink your tea. Feel free to enhance the palate of plain water. Makes:1 Prep Time: 5 Mins Cook Time: 5 Mins Total Time: 13 Mins Calorie: 101kcal

8. Sirt Muesli

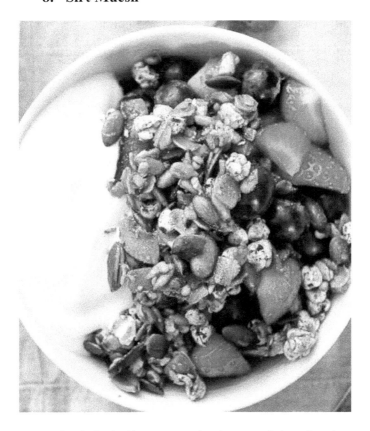

To make it in bulk or to make it overnight, simply put the dry ingredients together and store it in a container. Only apply the strawberries and yogurt the next day, and it's ready to go.

Ingredients:

- ✓ 10g buckwheat puffs

- ✓ 20g buckwheat flakes
- ✓ 100g strawberries, hulled and chopped
- ✓ 15g coconut flakes or desiccated coconut
- ✓ 15g walnuts, chopped
- ✓ 40g Medjool dates, pitted and chopped
- ✓ 10g cocoa nibs
- ✓ 100g plain Greek yogurt (or vegan alternative, such as soya or coconut yogurt)

Instructions:

Put together all of these products (leave the fruits and yogurt out if you don't instantly serve).

Makes:10 Prep Time: 10 Mins Cook Time: 25 Mins Total Time: 35 Mins Calorie: 211kcal

9. Matcha With Vanilla

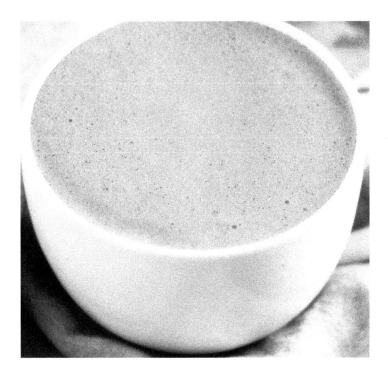

Swap the tasty green matcha and the white tea in this Japanese-style tea or coffee. It's easy to make at home, and it only takes 5 minutes

Ingredients:

- ✓ seeds from half a vanilla pod
- ✓ ½ tsp matcha powder

Instruction:

✓ Heat the kettle then apply 100ml of water to it. In a tiny cup, pour half the hot tea, steam and then transfer the matcha powder and vanilla seeds to the remainder of the bottle.

✓ Stir the mixture up to a smooth, slightly smooth and lump-free matcha with a bamboo whisk or mini-electric whisk. In a hot teapot, throw the water away and then dump the cooked matcha tea into it.

Makes:1mug Prep Time: 5 Mins Cook Time: 5 Mins Total Time: 10 Mins

10. Turmeric Tea

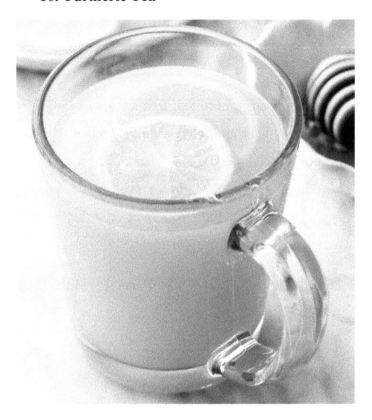

Take the spice rack and catch turmeric to create this coffee-free drink. This orange spice occurs everywhere on the menus

Ingredients:

- ✓ 1 tbsp fresh grated ginger
- ✓ 3 heaped tsp ground turmeric

✓ honey or agave and lemon slices, to serve

✓ One small orange, zest pared

Instructions:

✓ Boil in a pot 500ml of tea. Into a teapot or jug, put turmeric, ginger and orange-pink. Sprinkle with the heating water for about 5 minutes.

✓ Strain into two cups using a sieve or Tea strainer, apply a slice of lemon and sweeten, whether you prefer, with sweet honey or agave.

Makes:2 Prep Time: 5 Mins Cook Time: 15 Mins Total Time: 15 Mins

12. Date And Walnut Cinnamon Bites

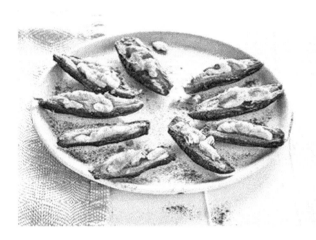

These cinnamon dates and walnut bites are quick to whip for a good snack. They act even as a reward when you have friends

Ingredients:

- ✓ Three pitted Medjool dates
- ✓ Three walnut halves
- ✓ Add the ground cinnamon, to taste

Instruction:

✓ Split each walnut half carefully into three pieces and then do the same with the dates. Place on top of every date a piece of walnut and cover with cinnamon dust.

Makes:1 Prep Time: 5 Mins Cook Time: 0 Mins Total Time: 5 Mins Calorie: 168kcal

13. Red Chicory, Pear And Hazelnut Salad

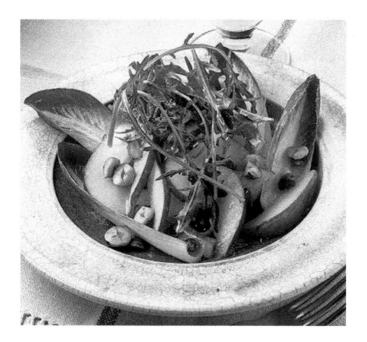

Ingredients:

- ✓ For the dressing
- ✓ 1 tsp sherry or cider vinegar
- ✓ Two heads of red chicory or white if not available
- ✓ 25g hazelnuts, toasted and chopped
- ✓ Two ripe red Williams pears a good handful of rocket leaves
- ✓ 2 tbsp hazelnut or olive oil
- ✓ 1 tsp green peppercorns in brine, optional
- ✓ 2 tbsp. of salad oil, either sunflower oil or oil with safflower.

Instructions:

- ✓ Dress up. If they use green pepper beans, lightly crush them in a bowl or use a pestle and mortar with a wooden spoon. Mix the oils and vinegar and sprinkle with the salt.
- ✓ Remove the stalk from the chicory and remove any cute or tired external leaves. Break the leaves carefully and organize 5-6 in 4 sections-whether each one is big, cut or tear.

- ✓ Take the tongs out of the pears, and lengthwise quarter the pears. Cut the kernel and dice the fruit thinly. Arrange the chicory slices and spoon more than half of the sauce. Pour over the rocket the remaining dressing and salt and pepper season. Place the leaves on top of each salad and easily flip. Sprinkle and top with almonds.

Makes: 2 servings Prep Time: 15 Mins Cook Time: 0 Mins Total Time: 15 Mins Calorie: 174kcal

14. Italian Kale

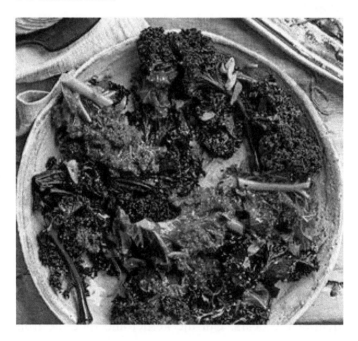

This vibrant green lateral dish was tasted and dressing in vinegar, giving it a sweet and sour taste, which keeps you coming back for longer.

Ingredients:

- ✓ Three tbsp red wine vinegar
- ✓ Three garlic cloves, finely sliced
- ✓ Three tbsp olive oil
- ✓ 300g cavolo nero or kale, roughly shredded

Instructions:

- ✓ Then apply the vinegar and a splash of water to heat the oil into a large bowl with a plate, fill it with garlic.
- ✓ Top up the kale and cover the steam, adding more water if the pot gets too dry for 4-5 minutes. Season with a little salt of the sea once wilted.

Makes:4 servings Prep Time: 5 Mins Cook Time: 5 Mins Total Time: 10 Mins Calorie: 50kcal

15. Broccoli And Kale Green Soup

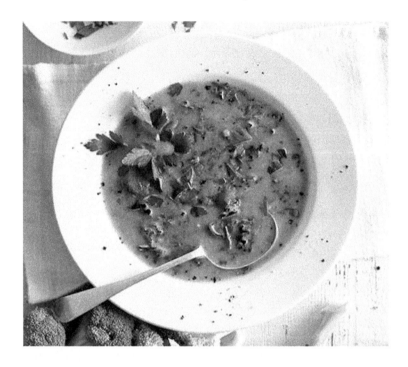

This super healthy soup combines broccoli with ginger, coriander and turmeric to make a dense and fat lunch with nutrients.

Ingredients:

- ✓ One tbsp sunflower oil
- ✓ 500ml, by mixing powder of 1 tbsp broth and boiling water in a jug
- ✓ Two garlic cloves, sliced

- ✓ Sliced ½ tsp ground coriander, thumb-sized piece ginger.
- ✓ Piece 3 cm / 1 in the fresh, fresh root of turmeric, peeled and grated or 1⁄2 tsp.
- ✓ 85g broccoli100g kale, chopped
- ✓ 200g courgettes, roughly sliced
- ✓ One lime, zested and juiced
- ✓ A thin, finely chopped parsley pack with a few whole leaves.

Instructions

- ✓ In a deep pot place the butter, add the garlic, ginger, coriander, salt and turmeric, fry over medium heat for 2 minutes, then add 3 tbsp of water, give the spices a little more moisture.
- ✓ Add the courgettes, ensure that the slices have a good mixture of all the spices, then cook 3 minutes. Add stock of 400 ml and cook for 3 minutes.
- ✓ Add the remaining stock to the broccoli, kale and lime juice. Let all vegetables soft and cook once more for 3-4 minutes.
- ✓ Remove the heat and add the pickled parsley. Load it all into a machine and blend it easily to high speed.

It'll be a pretty leaf with patches of shadow (the kale). Decorate with parsley and lime.

Makes:2 servings Prep Time: 15 Mins Cook Time: 20 Mins Total Time: 35 Mins Calorie: 182kcal

16. Strawberry, Tomato And Watercress Salad With Honey & Pink Pepper Dressing

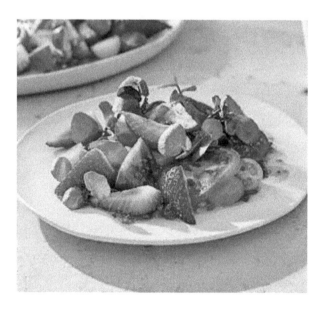

As a side meal, or even for lunch on your own, eat this cherry, tomato and aquarel salad. Pink peppers offer a gentle spice in the dressing

Ingredients:

- ✓ 100g watercress, woody stalks discarded
- ✓ 300g strawberries
- ✓ Three tbsp extra virgin olive oil
- ✓ Two strawberries (about 40g), chopped
- ✓ For the dressing
- ✓ Three tbsp pink peppercorns
- ✓ ½ lemon, juiced
- ✓ ½ tbsp honey
- ✓ 250g mixed tomatoes

Instructions:

- ✓ Toast the potatoes with a dry pot for 1-2 minutes, then cook quickly with a stick and a touch of Salt to split up the skins.
- ✓ To prepare the sauce. Attach and crush the two strawberries into a paste.
- ✓ Stir in the lemon juice and the honey. In a large bowl, put the dressing and the olive oil whisk. Please check

the seasoning and if you like, add a bit more salt or lemon juice. To assemble the bowl, split the strawberries into quarters or thin wedges, and finely slice the tomatoes, chopping some and halving others, so you get plenty of various shapes. In the bowl, mix with the hammer.

✓ Place the salad on a tray, or layer the salad between four pots. Spoon over the left clothes in the tub.

Makes:2 servings Prep Time: 10 Mins Cook Time: 2 Mins Total Time: 12 Mins Calorie: 128kcal

17. Oriental Salmon And Broccoli Traybake

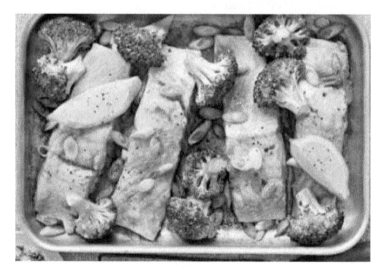

Everything you need to create this Asian flavored fish dish with balanced greens and fresh lemon is five ingredients

Ingredients:

- ✓ One head broccoli, broken into florets
- ✓ Four skin-on salmon fillets
- ✓ juice ½ lemon, ½ lemon quartered
- ✓ Two tbsp soy sauce
- ✓ small bunch spring onions, sliced

Instructions:

- ✓ 180C/160C heating stove/gas 4. Place the salmon in a large tin of roasts, making space for each fillet.
- ✓ Wash and dry broccoli and arrange around the fillets, while still a little wet. Place overall the lemon water, then apply the quarter of a lemon.
- ✓ Sprinkle half the onions with a little olive oil and add them to the oven for 14 minutes. Sprinkle it with the soy, detach from the oven, return for another 4 minutes to the oven before salmon is fried. Just before serving, sprinkle with the remaining spring onions.

Makes:2 servings Prep Time: 10 Mins Cook Time: 20 Mins
Total Time: 30 Mins Calorie: 310kcal

18. Superhealthy Salmon Salad

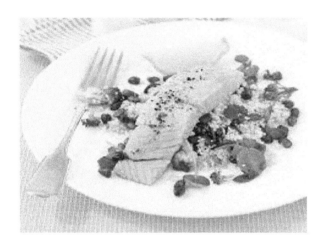

Super-healthy by word, super-healthy by nature: This salad
is rich in omega-3, iron and calcium and counts as 2 of your
five a day salad.

Ingredients:

- ✓ Two salmon fillets
- ✓ 100g couscous
- ✓ 1 tbsp olive oil

- ✓ juice one lemon
- ✓ 200g sprouting broccoli, roughly shredded, larger stalks removed
- ✓ a small handful of pumpkin seeds
- ✓ seeds from half a pomegranate
- ✓ Two handfuls watercress
- ✓ olive oil and extra lemon wedges, to serve

Instruction:

- ✓ Heat a stage steamer with gas. Season the couscous, then sprinkle with 1 tsp oil. Pour water over the couscous and cover it by 1 cm, then set aside. When the water in the steamer hits the simmer, tip the broccoli into the water and then place the salmon in the above stage—Cook for 3 minutes before the salmon is finished, and tender broccoli. Drain the broccoli and refrigerate under the cool spray.
- ✓ Add the remaining oil and lemon juice together. Toss the broccoli, pomegranate seeds and the pumpkin seeds with the lemon dressing through the couscous. Chop the watercress loosely at the last minute, then throw into the couscous. Serve, if you want, with the

tuna, lemon wedges to squeeze over and fresh olive oil to drizzle.

Makes:2 servings Prep Time: 20 Mins Cook Time: 5 Mins Total Time: 25 Mins Calorie: 320kcal

19. Malabar Prawns

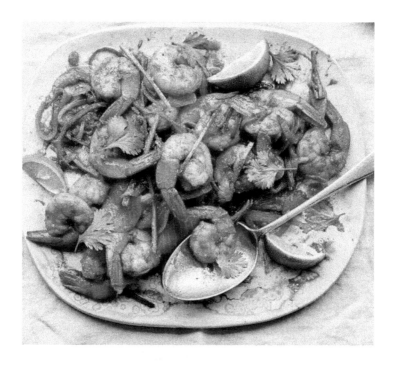

Create one of the favorite dishes of Kerala-Malabar prawns, a South Indian coast specialty. They are fast and easy to prepare and filled with distinct flavors

Ingredients:

- ✓ 400 grams of frozen king prawns2 tsp turmeric
- ✓ Kashmiri chili powder 3-4 tsp.
- ✓ Lemon juice of 4 tsp, with a pinch
- ✓ 40gm ginger, half peeled and dried, half finely cut in similar lines
- ✓ Vegetable oil 1 tbsp
- ✓ Four Leaves of curry
- ✓ Two - Four orange, half and desirable chilies
- ✓ One fine-sliced onion
- ✓ One tsp black pepper cracked
- ✓ 40gm new rubbed coconut
- ✓ 1⁄2 batch of coriander, leaves only

Instructions:

- ✓ Wash the prawns in cold water, then dry pick. Toss them and put aside with the turmeric, chili powder, lemon juice, and grated ginger.

✓ Heat the oil in a saucepan and add the curry leaves, chili, ginger sliced and onion. Cook for around 10 mins until translucent, then apply the black pepper.

✓ Stir-fry the prawns with some marinade once tender, around 2 minutes. Season and apply a squeeze of lemon juice if necessary. Serve with coconut and leaves of coriander added.

Makes:4 servings Prep Time: 15 Mins Cook Time: 12 Mins Total Time: 30 Mins Calorie: 422kcal

20. Chicken, Kale And Sprout Stir-Fry

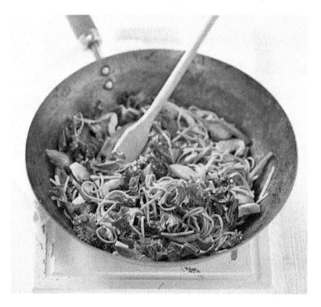

Brussels sprouts are not enough for Christmas-add them for extra protein and crunch in a balanced noodle dish

Ingredients:

- ✓ 100 g noodle soba.
- ✓ 100 g curly shredded broccoli.
- ✓ Sesame Oil 2 tsp.
- ✓ Two lean breasts of meat, skin off, cut into thin pieces.
- ✓ 25 g fresh ginger portion, peeled and cut into matching rods.
- ✓ One hot, required, thin-sliced pepper
- ✓ Handful sprouting of Brussels, sliced into pieces.
- ✓ One tbsp of soy sauce low sodium
- ✓ 2 tbsp rice wine or vinegar with white wine
- ✓ One lime juice and zest.

Instructions:

- ✓ Cook the noodles according to the directions for packaging, then drain and set aside. In the meantime, heat a large wok or frying pan and add the kale with a good splash of water and cook for 1-2 minutes until wild, with the remaining snap, then cool under running water to keep the color.

✓ Add half the oil and cook the chicken strips until browned, then cut and put differently. Heat the remaining oil until it is a little softened, cook the ginger, pepper and sprout. Remove the poultry and kale and add the noodles.

✓ Tip on the soy, rice wine, lime zest and juice along with enough water to make a sauce that adheres to ingredients, serve straight away.

Makes:2 servings Prep Time: 10 Mins Cook Time: 20 Mins Total Time: 30 Mins Calorie: 390kcal

21. Chicken, Broccoli And Beetroot Salad With Avocado Pesto

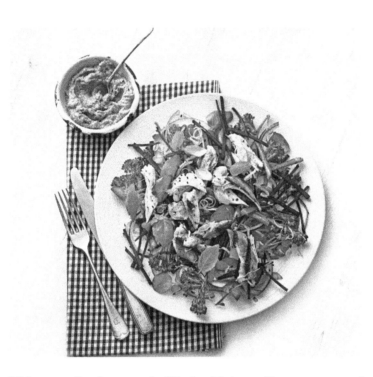

This superfood supper is filled with ingredients to strengthen the body, including red onion, rapeseed oil, nigella seeds, walnuts, and lemon

Ingredients:

- ✓ Thin-strained broccoli 250gm.
- ✓ Rapeseed oil 2 tsp.

- ✓ Three skinless breasts of chicken.
- ✓ One red thinly sliced onion.
- ✓ Watercress 100g bag.
- ✓ Two raw beetroots (about 175 g), peeled
- ✓ Seeds of nigella 1 tsp.
- ✓ For pesto avocado.
- ✓ Small basil bag.
- ✓ One Avocado.
- ✓ Smashed 1/2 garlic cloves
- ✓ Crumbled 25 g walnut pieces
- ✓ Rapeseed oil 1 tbsp.
- ✓ One lemon juice and zest.

Instructions:

- ✓ Bring to a boil a wide pan of water, add the broccoli and cook for 2 minutes. Drain, then under cool water to clean. Heat a griddle plate, toss the broccoli for 2-3 mins in 1/2 tsp of the rapeseed oil and griddle, rotating, until a little charred. Put aside to freshen up. Brush the remaining oil and season into the bird. Griddle on either side for 3-4 minutes or until it is cooked clean. Leave to cool, then break into chunky bits or shred them.

✓ Insert the pesto next. Choose the basil leaves, then set aside a few of them to cover the salad. Place the remainder inside a food processor's little pot. Scoop the avocado flesh and add the garlic, walnuts, sugar, 1 tbsp lemon juice, 2-3 tbsp of cold water and some seasoning to the food processor. Blitz until flat, then move to a small serving platter. Pour the remainder of the lemon juice over the sliced onions, and leave for a few minutes.

✓ Put the watercress onto a broad bowl. Toss the broccoli and onion, along with the lemon juice in which they were soaked. Top up the beetroot, but don't combine it with the chicken. Disperse the reserved basil leaves, lemon zest and nigella seeds and serve with pesto avocado.

Makes:4 servings Prep Time: 15 Mins Cook Time: 15 Mins Total Time: 30 Mins Calorie: 320kcal

22. Kale With Lemon Tahini Dressing

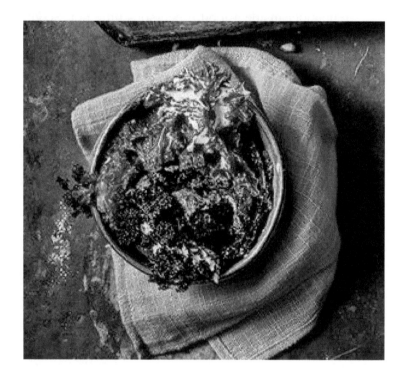

A simple and easy side dish stir-fried on the kale. Drizzle over a glug of the lemon tahini dressing to make your greens flavourful and new

Ingredients:

- ✓ One lemon juice (about 3 tbsp)
- ✓ Smashed One garlic clove.
- ✓ Tahini 50 g.

- ✓ One cup of olive oil.
- ✓ Kale 200 g.

Instructions:

- ✓ Next, button it up. In a tiny cup, apply the lemon juice, garlic, tahini and 50ml of cool water. Mix well to shape a loose dressing and to taste the season. (Don't panic if it gets divided at first – it should fall back when you mix it).
- ✓ Heat the oil in a big pot and stir-fry the kale for 3 minutes. Attach half the dressing to the saucepan and cook for 30 secs. Move the remaining dressing to a serving bowl and drizzle over.

Makes:2 servings Prep Time: 5 Mins Cook Time: 5 Mins Total Time: 10 Mins Calorie: 274kcal

23. The Sirtfood Diet's Coronation Chicken Salad

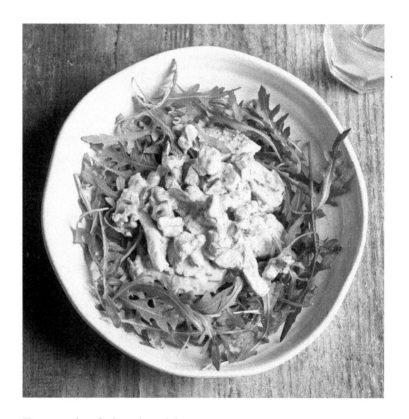

Easy and safe lunch-spirits

Ingredients:

- ✓ 75 g Yogurt Regular
- ✓ 1/4th lemon water
- ✓ One tablespoon, chopped, coriander

- ✓ One tablespoon. Turmeric field
- ✓ 1/2 tablespoon of mild curry powder
- ✓ 100 g Cooked breast chicken, sliced into bite-size
- ✓ 6 Half walnut, finely minced
- ✓ 1 Date of Medjool, thinly cut
- ✓ 20 g Dice of red onion
- ✓ 1 Chili bird's eye
- ✓ Rocket 40 grams, for eating

Instructions:

- ✓ In a mug, mix the yogurt, lemon juice, coriander and spices. Attach the remainder of the ingredients and put on a rocket pad.

Makes:1 serving Prep Time: 0 Mins Cook Time: 5 Mins Total Time: 5 Mins Calorie: 105kcal

24. The Sirtfood Diet's Bunless Beef Burgers With All The Trimmings

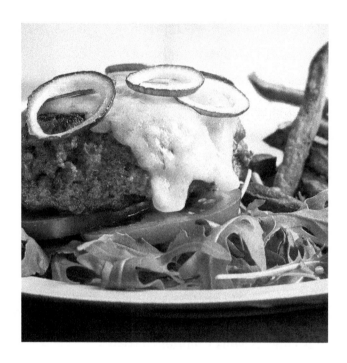

Everybody likes a good burger with sweet fries

Ingredients:

- ✓ 125 g of lean minced beef (5% fat)
- ✓ 15 g of red, finely diced onion.
- ✓ One tablespoon of Parsley, diced thinly
- ✓ One tablespoon of Extra virgin Olive oil

- ✓ Sweet potatoes 150 g
- ✓ One tablespoon of Olive oil super-pure
- ✓ One tablespoon of clean rosemary
- ✓ 1 Clove of garlic, unpeeled
- ✓ 10 gm Cheese cheddar, cut or grated
- ✓ 150 g red, ring-sliced onion
- ✓ 30 gm Sliced tomato
- ✓ Missile weighing 10 gm
- ✓ One (optional) Gherkin

Instructions:

- ✓ Heat the oven up to 220oC / gas 7
- ✓ Start by making some fries. Peel and shape into 1 cm thick chips the sweet potato. Attach the olive oil, rosemary and garlic clove to them. Place on a baking sheet and fry for 30 minutes, until smooth and crisp.
- ✓ For the steak, combine the ground beef with the onion and the parsley. Unless you have pastry cutters, you may be able to shape your burger with the biggest pastry cutter in the package, otherwise, use your hands to create only a decent patty.

✓ Heat the frying pan over medium heat, add the oil, put the burger on one side of the pan and rings the onion on the other side. Cook the burger on each side for 6 minutes, to ensure it is cooked through. When fried to your taste, fry the onion rings.

✓ Top with the cheese and red onion when the burger is cooked and place it in a hot oven for a minute to melt. Remove the tomato, rocket and gherkin and top it with. Serve with some fries.

Makes:1 servings Prep Time: 15 Mins Cook Time: 30 Mins Total Time: 45 Mins Calorie: 385kcal

25. The Sirtfood Diet's Chicken Skewers With Satay Sauce

Dinner with minimal effort, full of taste and spice

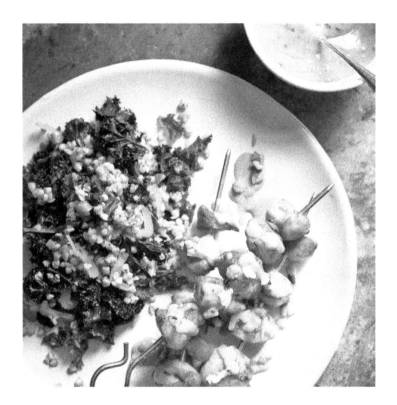

Ingredients:

- ✓ 150 g of chicken breast, cut into pieces.
- ✓ One tablespoon terrestrial turmeric.
- ✓ 1/2 tablespoon live oil is particularly virgin.

- ✓ Buckwheat: 50 g.
- ✓ Kale 30 g, stalks removed and trimmed.
- ✓ 30 gm Sliced celery.
- ✓ Four half walnut, sliced, to garnish.
- ✓ 20 g diced red onion
- ✓ One Clove of garlic, minced
- ✓ One tablespoon olive oil is particularly virgin
- ✓ One tablespoon curried milk
- ✓ One tablespoon terrestrial turmeric
- ✓ Chicken stock: 50 ml
- ✓ Coconut milk: 150 ml
- ✓ 1tablespoon butter with walnut or peanut butter
- ✓ One tablespoon chopped Coriander

Instructions:

- ✓ mix the chicken with olive oil and turmeric and reserve to marinate-30 minutes to 1 hour is best, but just leave it as long as you can if you are short in time.
- ✓ Cook the buckwheat and add the kale and celery to the last 5–7 minutes of the cooking time according to the package instructions. Hey, drain.
- ✓ Heat the barbecue in a high setting.

72

- ✓ Gently fry the red onion and garlic in the olive oil for 2-3 minutes until soft. Add the spices and cook for another minute. Add the stock and the coconut milk and bring to a boil, then add the walnut butter and stir. Reduce heat and simmer the sauce for 8-10 minutes or until creamy and rich.
- ✓ As the sauce simmers, add the chicken to the skewers and place it under the hot grill for 10 minutes, turning it after 5 minutes.
- ✓ To serve, stir the coriander in the sauce and pour over the skewers, then spread over the chopped walnuts.

Makes:1 servings Prep Time: 10 Mins Cook Time: 30 Mins Total Time: 40 Mins Calorie: 365kcal

26. The Sirtfood Diet's Smoked Salmon Omelette

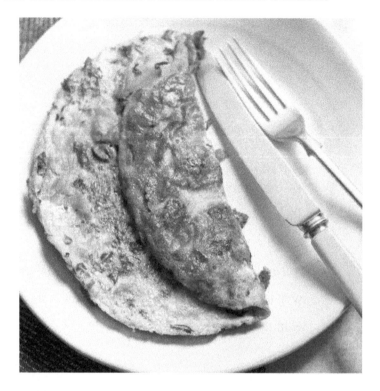

Try this quick and easy Sirtfood dish, packed with taste and goodness.

Makes: 1, Prep Time: 0 Hours 5 Mins, Cook Time: 0 Hours 0 Mins, Total Time: 0 Hours 5 Mins

Ingredients:

- ✓ Two eggs small
- ✓ 100 g Smoked, cut salmon

- ✓ 1/2 dc. Capers.-Capers
- ✓ 10 g of a rocket, cut
- ✓ One tablespoon chopped Parsley
- ✓ One tablespoon olive oil extra virgin

Instructions:

- ✓ Smash the eggs and whisk them into a tub. Stir in the salmon, capers, rockets, and Persil.
- ✓ In a non-stick oven, heat the olive oil till it is dry, but not smoking. Attach the egg blend and push the blend around the pan using a spatula or fish slice until even. Reduce the heat and cook the omelet. Slide around the edges of the spatula and roll the omelet or fold it in half to serve.

Makes:1 servings Prep Time: 5 Mins Cook Time: 5 Mins Total Time: 10 Mins Calorie: 275kcal

27. The Sirtfood Diet's Shakshuka

Enjoy this spicy fried egg and kale recipe.

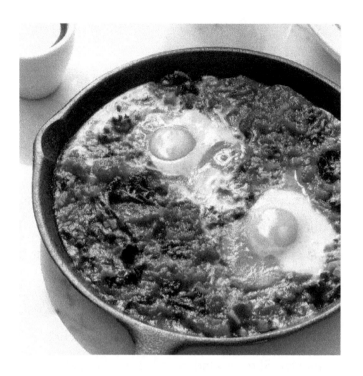

Ingredients:

- ✓ One tablespoon of olive Oil Extra Virgin
- ✓ 40 gm of fine cut red onion
- ✓ One Garlic clove, thinly sliced
- ✓ Thirty grams of celery, chopped
- ✓ Chili 1 bird's eye, good cut
- ✓ One tablespoon cumin Groud
- ✓ One tablespoon turmeric – Field turmeric.
- ✓ One tablespoon paprika.
- ✓ 400 g Chopped tinned tomatoes

✓ 30 g Kale, trimmed stalks and cut roughly.

✓ One tablespoon Parsley captured.

✓ Two small eggs.

Instructions:

✓ Heat over medium to low heat a small, deep-seated frying pan. Add the oil and fry for 1–2 minutes onion, garlic, celery, chili, and spices.

✓ Add the tomatoes, then leave the sauce for 20 minutes to heat slowly, stirring periodically.

Makes:1 servings Prep Time: 0 Mins Cook Time: 40 Mins Total Time: 40 Mins Calorie: 280kcal

28. The Sirtfood Diet's Date And Walnut Porridge

Get a great start to the day with this Sirtfood breakfast

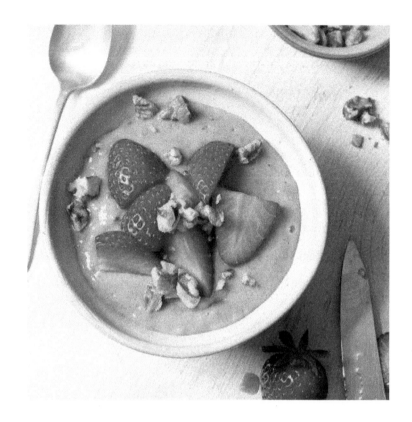

Ingredients:

- ✓ 50 g Strawberries, hulled
- ✓ 200 ml Milk or dairy-free alternative
- ✓ 35 g Buckwheat flakes
- ✓ One Medjool date, chopped
- ✓ One tsp. Walnut butter or four chopped walnut halves

Instructions:

- ✓ Put the milk and the date in a saucepan, heat gently, then add the buckwheat flakes and cook until the porridge is the consistency you like.
- ✓ Add the walnut butter or walnuts, stir in the strawberries and serve.
- ✓ Mix in the kale and roast for another 5 minutes. When you thought the sauce is too deep, just apply a bit of water. Stir in the parsley, if your sauce has a good rich flavor.
- ✓ Make two small sauce wells and spit each egg into them. Reduce heat to its lowest setting and use a lid or foil to cover the pan. Leave the eggs for 10–12 minutes to cook, where the whites should be firm while the yolks are still runny. Cook for an extra 3–4 minutes, if you like strong yolks. Serve right away-preferably straight from the jar.

Makes:1 servings Prep Time: 0 Mins Cook Time: 10 Mins Total Time: 10 Mins Calorie: 180kcal

29. The Sirtfood Diet's Braised Puy Lentils

This slow-roasted recipe is full of flavor

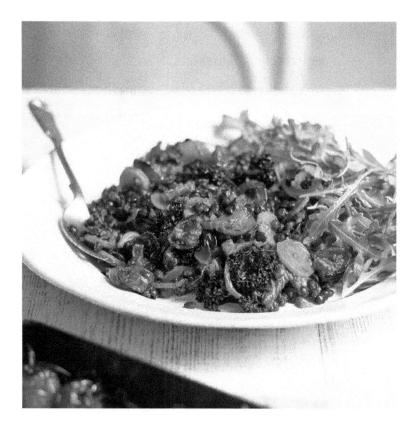

Ingredients:

- ✓ 8 Cherry tomatoes halved
- ✓ 40 g Red onion, thinly sliced
- ✓ 2 tsp. Extra virgin olive oil
- ✓ 40 g Celery, thinly sliced

- ✓ 1 Garlic clove, finely chopped
- ✓ 1 tsp. Paprika
- ✓ 40 g Carrots, peeled and thinly sliced
- ✓ 1 tsp. Thyme (dry or fresh)
- ✓ 220 ml Vegetable stock
- ✓ 75 g Puy lentils
- ✓ 20 g Rocket
- ✓ 1 tbsp. Parsley, chopped
- ✓ 50 g Kale, roughly chopped

Instructions:

- ✓ Heat up 120 ° C / gas 1/2. Heat your oven.
- ✓ In a small roasting tin, place the tomatoes and roast in the oven for 35-45 minutes.
- ✓ Heat the bowl over a medium-low flame. Stir the red Onion, garlic, celery and carotene in 1 teaspoon of olive oil, fry it for 1–2 minutes, until softened. Attach the paprika and thyme and cook for a minute.
- ✓ Rinse the lenses and add them to the pot along with the stock in a finely mixed pan. Bring to boil, then raising heat and cook with a cloth on the saucepan for 20 minutes. Add a little water if

the level drops too much and add a stir every 7 minutes.

✓ Cook for another 10 minutes, add the kale. Stir in the pettles and roasted tomatoes when the lentils are cooked. Serve the remaining tablespoon with the olive oil with the racket. Serve.

Makes:1 servings Prep Time: 40 Mins Cook Time: 0 Mins Total Time: 40 Mins Calorie: 90kcal

30. The Sirtfood Diet's Prawn Arrabbiata

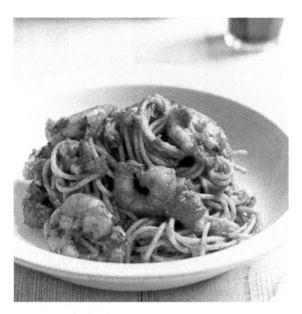

Ingredients:

- ✓ 65 g Buckwheat pasta
- ✓ Raw or cooked prawns (Ideally king prawns)
- ✓ One tbsp of Extra virgin olive oil
- ✓ One Garlic clove, finely chopped
- ✓ 40 g Red onion, finely chopped
- ✓ 1 Bird's eye chili, finely chopped
- ✓ 30 g Celery, finely chopped
- ✓ 1 tsp. Dried mixed herbs
- ✓ 1 tsp. Extra virgin olive oil
- ✓ 400 g Tinned chopped tomatoes
- ✓ 2 tbsp. White wine (optional)
- ✓ 1 tbsp. Chopped parsley

Instructions:

- ✓ Fry in oil for a half-low heat and for 1-2 minutes the onion, garlic, celery and chili and herbs. Turn the heat to moderate, add the wine for 1 minute and cook. Attach tomatoes and keep the sauce cooled for 20-30 minutes over medium-low heat until the sauce is nice and creamy. Just add a little water if you feel the sauce becomes too thick.
- ✓ Carry a bowl of water to boil during cooking and cook the pasta as instructed by the packet. Drain the

olive oil and hold in the pan until required when cooked to your taste.

- ✓ Add raw creams to the sauce, cook for 3 to 4 minutes and then add the parsley until they have become rose and opaque, and serve. Bring the sauce to the boil and serve if you use cooked creams with parsley.
- ✓ Add to the sauce cooked pasta, carefully yet gently mix and serve.

Makes:1 servings Prep Time: 35 Mins Cook Time: 20 Mins Total Time: 55 Mins Calorie: 205kcal

31. The Sirtfood Diet's Turmeric Baked Salmon

Eastern spices, an easy and healthy dinner

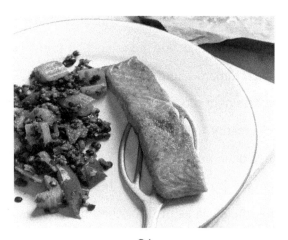

Ingredients:

- ✓ One tsp. Ground turmeric
- ✓ One tsp. Extra virgin olive oil
- ✓ One tsp. Extra virgin olive oil
- ✓ 1/4 Juice of a lemon
- ✓ 60 g Tinned green lentils
- ✓ 40 g Red onion, finely chopped
- ✓ One Bird's eye chili, finely chopped
- ✓ One Garlic clove, finely chopped
- ✓ One tsp. Mild curry powder
- ✓ 150 gm Celery, cut into 2cm lengths
- ✓ 100 ml Chicken or vegetable stock
- ✓ 130 gm Tomato, cut into eight wedges
- ✓ Skinned Salmon
- ✓ One tbsp. Chopped parsley

Instructions:

- ✓ Heat the oven to level 6 with gas / 200C.
- ✓ Start with the celery spicy. Heat a pot over moderate to low heat, add the onion, garlic, ginger, chili, and celery to the olive oil.

✓ Cook gently until soft and uncolored for about two to three minutes, then add the curry powder and start cooking for another minute.

✓ Add the tomatoes and the lenses and gently cook for about 10 minutes. You may want to increase or reduce the cooking time according to how crunchy the celery is.

✓ Mix turmeric, olive oil and lemon juice in the meantime. Cook for 8-10 minutes, place on a baking tray.

✓ Finish by mixing the celery with the silk and serving with the salmon.

Makes:1 servings Prep Time: 10 Mins Cook Time: 20 Mins Total Time: 30 Mins Calorie: 165kcal

32. Easy Peasy Chicken Curry

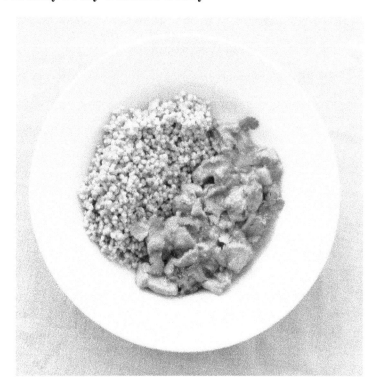

Ingredients

- ✓ Three garlic cloves roughly chopped
- ✓ One red onion roughly chopped
- ✓ Two teaspoons garam masala
- ✓ 2 cm fresh ginger peeled and roughly chopped
- ✓ Two teaspoons ground turmeric
- ✓ Two teaspoons ground cumin
- ✓ One cinnamon stick optional

- ✓ One tbsp of olive oil
- ✓ Six cardamom pods optional
- ✓ One x 400ml tin coconut milk
- ✓ Eight boneless of chicken thighs, cut into bitesize chunks, or four chicken breasts.
- ✓ 200 gm of brown or basmati rice buckwheat to dish.
- ✓ Two tablespoons fresh coriander chopped (plus extra for garnish)

Instructions:

- ✓ In the food processor, put the onion, garlic and ginger and lightning until the paste. Alternatively, chop these three ingredients thoroughly and continue as below, if you don't have one.
- ✓ Stir in the paste with the garam massale, cumin and turmeric. Place aside. Set aside.
- ✓ Placed in a big depth (ideally non-stick) 1 tablespoon of olive oil. For a minute, heat up the bowl, then add the chopped chicken thighs. Pour the chicken over high heat, and add to the curry paste. Turn it down for 2 minutes.

- ✓ Let the chicken cook for 3 minutes in the paste and then add half the milk (200ml) and the cinnamon (if using) cardamom. Turn down and cook until the curried sauce is thick and delicious, and then let it simmer for 30 minutes.
- ✓ Apply more coconut milk as the curry starts to heat, maybe you don't need anything, but if you want a much more clever curry, add the lot!
- ✓ Make your accompaniment (snack/rice) and any side dishes during the cooking process.
- ✓ When the curry is finished, add the sliced coriander and serve with sweet or rice and a good glass of chilled white wine, medium water immediately!

Makes:4 servings Prep Time: 15 Mins Cook Time: 30 Mins Total Time: 45 Mins Calorie: 165kcal

33. King Prawn Stir Fry With Buckwheat Noodles

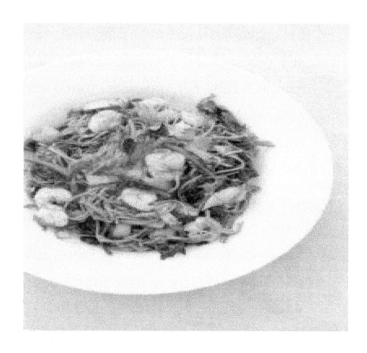

Ingredients:

- ✓ Two tablespoons extra virgin olive oil
- ✓ 300 g buckwheat/soba noodles try to get 100% buckwheat if you can
- ✓ Two sticks of celery sliced
- ✓ One red onion sliced thinly
- ✓ 100 g green beans chopped
- ✓ 100 g kale roughly chopped
- ✓ Three garlic cloves grated or finely chopped
- ✓ 3 cm ginger grated

- ✓ 600 g king prawns
- ✓ One bird's eye chili seeds/membranes removed and chopped finely (or more to taste)
- ✓ Two tablespoons tamari/soy sauce plus extra for serving
- ✓ Two tablespoons parsley chopped (or lovage if you can get it!)

Instructions:

- ✓ Cook noodles for 3-5 minutes or until you like them. Rinse in cold water, wash. Drizzle over a little olive oil, mix together and hold.
- ✓ Prepare remaining ingredients while the noodles are cooking.
- ✓ Fry the red onion and celery in a broad wok or saucepan for 3 minutes in moderate heat in a mild olive oil and add the kale and green boobs and cook for three minutes in medium-high heat.
- ✓ Remove heat and add ginger, garlic, chili and butter. Crumble for 2-3 minutes until crevasses are dry.
- ✓ Add noodles, tamari/soy sauce, and cook 1-minute longer until the noodles are again dry. Strain and serve with parsley.

Makes:1 servings Prep Time: 10 Mins Cook Time: 10 Mins
Total Time: 45 Mins Calorie: 185kcal

34. Baked Potatoes With Spicy Chickpea Stew (Vegan)

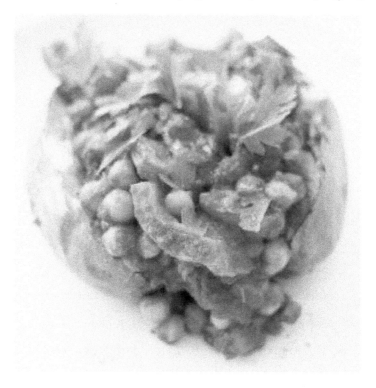

Spicy Chickpea Curry baked potatoes. Mexican mole kind
meets North African tagine. It's amazingly amazing, makes

a perfect top for baked pulp, as well as vegetarian, vegan, gluten-free and milk free. And the chocolate is there.

Ingredients:

- ✓ Two tablespoons olive oil
- ✓ 4-6 baking potatoes pricked all over
- ✓ Four cloves garlic grated or crushed
- ✓ Two red onions finely chopped
- ✓ 2 cm ginger grated
- ✓ Two tablespoons cumin seeds
- ✓ ½ -two tsp of chili flakes depending on how hot you like things
- ✓ Splash of water
- ✓ Two tablespoons turmeric
- ✓ Two tsp unsweetened cocoa powder or cacao
- ✓ 2 x 400g tins chickpeas or kidney beans if you prefer, including the chickpea water, don't drain!
- ✓ Two yellow peppers or whatever color you prefer! chopped into bitesize pieces
- ✓ 2 x 400g tins chopped tomatoes
- ✓ Salt and pepper to taste optional
- ✓ Two tablespoons parsley plus extra for garnish
- ✓ Side salad optional

Instructions:

- ✓ Preheat the oven to 200C, while all the ingredients can be prepared.
- ✓ Put the baking potatoes in the oven when the oven is hot enough, and cook 1 hour or until they're finished as you want them. (If it's different from mine, feel free to use your usual baked potato method!)
- ✓ Put olive oil and chopped red onion in an oven in a big broad casserole once in the oven and gradually cook with the lid until the onion is tender, but not brown for 5 minutes.
- ✓ Remove the lid and add the cumin, chili and garlic. Add the curds and a very small splash of water for another minute and cook for a minute, taking care not to let the pan dry enough and cook for a minute.
- ✓ Add the tomatoes and cacao powder, chickpeas and yellow pepper, as well as chickpea juice. Bring to a boil, then cook 45 minutes on low heat until the sauce is thick and unctuous (but do not

allow it to burn!). The stew will take place roughly with the potatoes.

✓ Serve a skewer with a simple side salad on the baked Pommes of terracotta, and add 2 table cubs of parsley, salt and pepper if necessary.

Makes:4 servings Prep Time: 10 Mins Cook Time: 60 Mins Total Time: 1 hour 10 Mins Calorie: 500kcal

35. Kale And Red Onion Dhal With Buckwheat (Vegan)

Kale and Buckwheat Red Onion Dhal. This Kale and Red Onion Dhal are delicious and very nutritious with buckwheat that can be conveniently and quickly processed without gluten, milk, vegetarians or vegan.

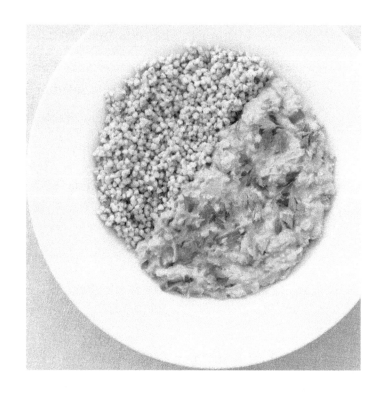

Ingredients:

- ✓ One small red onion sliced
- ✓ One tablespoon olive oil
- ✓ 2 cm ginger grated
- ✓ Three garlic cloves grated or crushed
- ✓ Two teaspoons turmeric
- ✓ One bird's eye chili deseeded and finely chopped (more if you like things hot!)
- ✓ 160 g red lentils

- ✓ Two teaspoons garam masala
- ✓ 200 ml of water
- ✓ 400 ml of coconut milk
- ✓ 160 g buckwheat or brown rice
- ✓ 100 g kale or spinach would be a great alternative

Instructions:

- ✓ In a deep, broad casserole, put the olive oil and add onion sliced. Cook in low heat and the lid will be softened for 5 minutes.
- ✓ Add garlic, chili-ginger and cook for another 1 minute.
- ✓ Attach the turmeric and a sprinkling of water to the garam masala, and cook for another 1 minute.
- ✓ Apply the red lens, chocolate milk and 200 ml water (just half of the cocoa milk can be filled with water and tipped into the cup).
- ✓ Mix everything carefully and cook over low heat with the lid for 20 minutes. Extract from time to time, add some more water if the dhal sticks.
- ✓ Stir and remove your cap, add kale after 20 minutes (1-2 minutes if you're wearing spinach instead!); cook for another 5 minutes.

✓ Put buckwheat in a medium pot and add plenty of boiling water about 15 minutes before the curry is ready. Return the water to the boil again and cook 10 minutes (or a little longer if it is softer. Drain the buckwheat into a sieve and use the dhal.

Makes:4 servings Prep Time: 5 Mins Cook Time: 25 Mins Total Time:30 Mins Calorie: 402kcal

36. The Sirtfood Diet Green Salad

Superb and simple to construct.

This salad includes two more Sirt, walnuts and olive oil with the same ingredients as the green drink, as well as the orange Sirt.

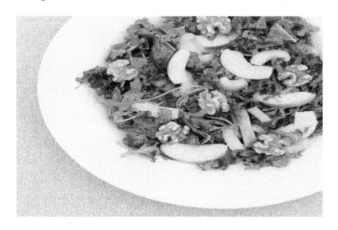

Ingredients:

- ✓ 1 cm of ginger grated
- ✓ Juice of ½ lemon
- ✓ One tablespoon olive oil
- ✓ Salt and pepper to taste
- ✓ One handful rocket
- ✓ Two handfuls kale sliced
- ✓ Two celery sticks sliced
- ✓ One tablespoon parsley
- ✓ Six walnut halves
- ✓ ½ green apple sliced

Instructions:

- ✓ In a jam container, add the lemon juice, ginger, salt, pumice and olive oil.
- ✓ In a large cup, place the kale and pour over the dressing. Wear the dressing for 1 minute to rub into the kale.
- ✓ Add the other ingredients and thoroughly blend together.

Makes:4 servings Prep Time: 10 Mins Cook Time: 0 Mins Total Time:10 Mins Calorie: 557kcal

37. The Sirtfood Diet Green Juice

The green juice is full of nutrient-rich Sirt foods, which are taken from the recipes in the Sirtfood Diet. This is ideal for those who want to get healthy, important to the Sirtfood Diet.

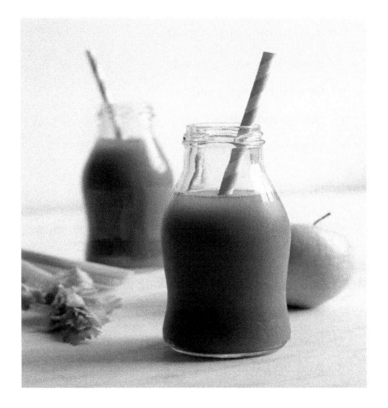

Ingredients:

✓ 30 g rocket

- ✓ 75 g kale
- ✓ 5 g parsley
- ✓ ½ green apple
- ✓ Two celery sticks
- ✓ Juice of ½ lemon
- ✓ 1 cm ginger
- ✓ ½ teaspoon matcha green tea

Instructions:

- ✓ Juice all the ingredients except the citrus and green tea matcha.
- ✓ Hand in the green juice squeeze the lemon juice
- ✓ Mix in a glass a tiny amount and add a little green juice. Through the bottle and add with the rest of the green juice.
- ✓ Save or drink immediately.

Makes:1 servings Prep Time: 5 Mins Cook Time: 0 Mins Total Time:5 Mins Calorie: 342kcal

38. Turmeric Chicken & Kale Salad With Honey Lime Dressing-Sirtfood Recipes

Notes: Dress the salad ten minutes before serving if prepared in advance. Beef small, chopped creeping prawns and fish can replace chicken. Vegetarians may use mushrooms or quinoa cooked.

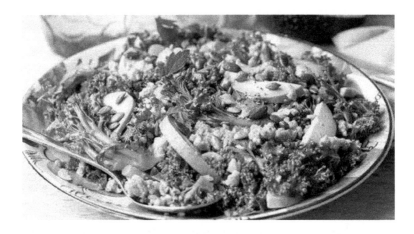

Ingredients:

For the chicken

- ✓ ½ medium brown onion, diced
- ✓ One tsp ghee or 1 tbsp of coconut oil
- ✓ One large garlic clove should be finely diced
- ✓ 250-300 g / 9 oz. chicken mince or diced up chicken thighs
- ✓ One teaspoon lime zest
- ✓ One teaspoon turmeric powder

- ✓ ½ teaspoon salt + pepper
- ✓ juice of ½ lime

For the salad

- ✓ Two tablespoons pumpkin seeds (pepitas)
- ✓ Six broccolini stalks or 2 cups of broccoli florets
- ✓ ½ avocado, sliced
- ✓ Three large kale leaves stem removed and chopped
- ✓ A handful of fresh parsley leaves, chopped
- ✓ A handful of fresh coriander leaves, chopped

For the dressing

- ✓ One small garlic clove, finely diced or grated
- ✓ Three tablespoons lime juice
- ✓ Three tablespoons extra-virgin olive oil (I used one tablespoon avocado oil and * 2 tablespoons EVO)
- ✓ One teaspoon raw honey
- ✓ Three tablespoons extra-virgin olive oil (I used one tablespoon avocado oil and * 2 tablespoons EVO)
- ✓ ½ teaspoon sea salt and pepper

- ✓ ½ teaspoon wholegrain or Dijon mustard

Instructions:

- ✓ In a small frying pan over medium to high flame, flame ghee or coconut oil. Add onion and sauté 4-5 minutes, until golden, at medium heat. Remove the chicken thin and garlic and brush over medium-high heat for 2-3 minutes and then separate.
- ✓ Mix and cook turmeric, lime zest, lime juice, salt and pepper for a further 3-4 minutes. Stir regularly. Put aside the cooked thin.
- ✓ Put a small pot of water to boil while the chicken is cooking. Stir and cook the broccolini for 2 minutes. Rince and cut into 3-4 pieces, each under cold water.
- ✓ Stirring regularly to avoid burning, add pumpkin seeds into the frypan from the chicken and toast over medium heat for 2 minutes. A little salt season. Season. Place aside. Set aside. Pure seeds from pumpkin are also appropriate for use.
- ✓ Place the sliced kale in a salad bowl and pipe over the sandwich. Place your hands on the dressing

and rub the egg. The sluts are smooth – they are partially "fried" – like citrus juice to fish or beef carpaccio. Bring in finally the fried rice, broccolini, new herbs, seeds of pumpkin and avocado.

Makes:1 servings Prep Time: 20 Mins Cook Time: 10 Mins Total Time:30 Mins Calorie: 282kcal

39. Buckwheat Noodles With Chicken Kale & Miso Dressing-Sirtfood Recipes

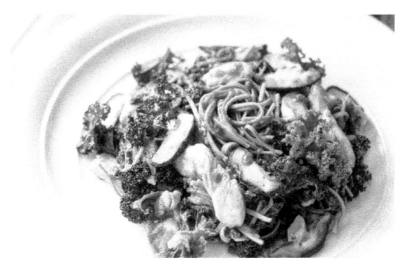

Ingredients:

For the noodles

- ✓ 2-3 pound of kale leaves (roughly cut out of the stem)
- ✓ Buckwheat noodles 150 g/5 oz (100% buckwheat, no wheat)
- ✓ 3-4 shiitake champagne, cut. Cut.
- ✓ One tablespoon of ghee or coconut oil
- ✓ One brown, fine-diced onion
- ✓ Chicken, sliced or diced one free-range media breast.
- ✓ One long, thinly sliced red chill (seeds inside or out, according to how hot you like)
- ✓ Two common, finely diced garlic cloves
- ✓ Tamari sauce with 2-3 teaspoons (gluten-free)

For the miso dressing

- ✓ One tablespoon Tamari sauce
- ✓ 1½ tablespoon fresh organic miso
- ✓ One tablespoon lemon or lime juice
- ✓ One tablespoon extra-virgin olive oil
- ✓ One teaspoon sesame oil (optional)

Instructions:

- ✓ Put to boil a medium water cup. Attach the kale and cook until slightly diluted, for 1 minute. Remove, save the water and bring it to the boil again. Drain it. Fill the soba noodles and cook (usually approximately 5 minutes) according to package directions. Rinse and set aside under cold water.
- ✓ Meanwhile, fry the shiitake champignon for 2-3 minutes with a little ghee or coconut oil (around a teaspoon), until nicely browned on either side. Pour in salt and set aside. Sprinkle.
- ✓ Heat coconut oil or ghee over medium-high heat in the same frying saucepan
- ✓ Pour into onion or chili and add chicken parts for 2-3 minutes. Cook over medium heat five minutes, stirring a few times, then add a small amount of garlic, tamari sauce, and tea. Cook for another 2-3 minutes, frequently mix until chicken is finished.
- ✓ Add the chicken noodle and soba, and cook up through the food.

✓ At the very end of cooking, blend the miso dressing and twinkling over the noodles to keep all of these beneficial probiotics alive.

Makes:1 servings Prep Time: 15 Mins Cook Time: 10 Mins Total Time:30 Mins Calorie: 405kcal

40. Choc Chip Granola-Sirtfood Recipes

Breakfast cake! Make sure to serve you plenty of SIRTs with a cup of green tea. If you want, you can substitute the rice malt syrup with maple syrup.

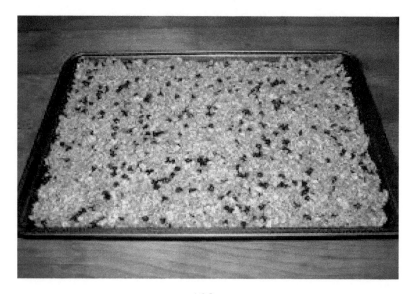

Ingredients:

- ✓ chopped
- ✓ 50g pecans, roughly
- ✓ 200g jumbo oats
- ✓ 20g butter
- ✓ 3 tbsp light olive oil
- ✓ 2 tbsp rice malt syrup
- ✓ 1 tbsp dark brown sugar
- ✓ dark chocolate chips
- ✓ 60g good-quality (70%)

Instructions

- ✓ Preheat oven to 140 ° C (gas 3). Preheat oven to 160 ° C. Line a major bakery with a sheet of silicone or pastry.
- ✓ In a large tub, mix oats and pecans. Heat olive oil, butter, brown sugar and rice malt syrup gently in a small, non-stick pot until butter melts and the sugar and syrup are dissolved. Don't authorize boiling. Pour the syrup over the oats

and mix until full coverage of the oats is complete.

✓ Spread the granola over the bakery and spread into the corners.

✓ Having mixture clumps with distance instead of spreading. Twenty minutes in the oven until the edges are light brown. Take out of the oven and allow the tray to refresh completely.

✓ Separate with your fingertips and then blend the chocolate with any large bumps in a tray when it's cold. Grab or pour the granola into a bowl or container airtight. At least two weeks the granola will stay.

Makes:2 servings Prep Time: 10 Mins Cook Time: 20 Mins Total Time:30 Mins Calorie: 350kcal

41. Baked Salmon Salad With Creamy Mint Dressing- Sirtfood Recipes

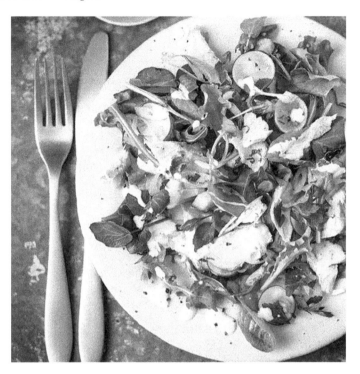

Ingredients:

- ✓ 40g mixed salad leaves
- ✓ One salmon fillet (130g)
- ✓ Two radishes, trimmed and thinly sliced
- ✓ 40g young spinach leaves
- ✓ Two spring onions, trimmed and sliced
- ✓ 5cm piece (50g) cucumber, cut into chunks

✓ One small handful (10g) parsley, roughly chopped

For the dressing:

✓ One tablespoon natural yogurt
✓ One tablespoon low-fat mayonnaise
✓ Two leaves mint, finely chopped
✓ One tablespoon rice vinegar
✓ Salt and freshly ground black pepper

Instructions:

✓ Preheat the oven to 200oC (fan/gas six at a temperature of 180oC).
✓ Through the salmon fillet on a baker and bake until cooked for 16-18 minutes. Remove and set aside from the oven. The salmon in the salad is just as nice warm or cold. If your salmon has meat, just cook the skin down and separate it from the skin with a fish slice. When fried, it will slide quickly.
✓ Mix the mayonnaise, yogurt and rice vinegar together in a small bowl and add the leaves and

salt and pepper with the mixture to allow the aromas to develop for at least 5 minutes.

- ✓ Settle the salad leaves and spinach with radishes, cucumber, ointments of the spring and pets on the serving plate and top. Place the cooked salmon on the salad and dress up.

Makes:1 servings Prep Time: 5 Mins Cook Time: 20 Mins Total Time:25 Mins Calorie: 340kcal

42. Fragrant Asian Hotpot-Sirtfood Recipes

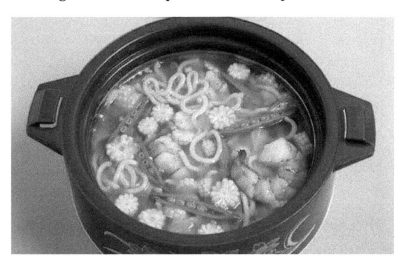

Ingredients:

- ✓ One star anise, crushed (or 1/4 tsp ground anise)

- ✓ 1 tsp tomato purée
- ✓ Small handful (10g) coriander, stalks finely chopped
- ✓ Small handful (10g) parsley, stalks finely chopped
- ✓ 1/2 carrot, peeled and cut into matchsticks
- ✓ 50gm beansprouts
- ✓ 50gm broccoli, cut into small florets
- ✓ 100gm firm tofu, chopped
- ✓ 100gm raw tiger prawns
- ✓ 50g rice noodles, cooked according to packet
- ✓ 20g sushi ginger, chopped
- ✓ 50g cooked water chestnuts, drained
- ✓ 1 tbsp good-quality miso paste

Instructions:

- ✓ Put in a bread pan and simmer for 10 minutes, the stirring tomato, star anise, petty stalks, coriander stalks and lime juice.
- ✓ Add carrot, broccoli, creeping pies, tofu, chestnuts and water noodles and gently cook until creeping is finished. Stir the sushi ginger and miso paste from the heat. Stir.

✓ Serve with pins and coriander leaves.

Makes:2 servings Prep Time: 5 Mins Cook Time: 10 Mins
Total Time:15 Mins Calorie: 185kcal

43. Lamb, Butternut Squash And Date Tagine-Sirtfood Recipes

Unbelievable dry Moroccan spices make this balanced day ideal for icy fall and winter days. For an extra health kick, serve with buckwheat!

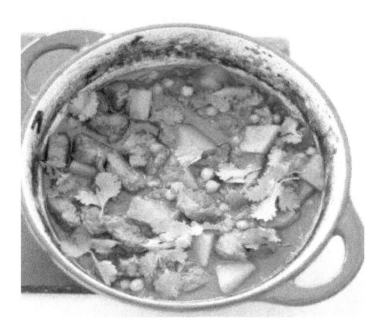

Ingredients:

- ✓ One red onion, sliced
- ✓ Two tablespoons olive oil
- ✓ Three garlic cloves, grated or crushed
- ✓ 2cm ginger, grated
- ✓ Two teaspoons cumin seeds
- ✓ One teaspoon chili flakes (or to taste)
- ✓ Two teaspoons ground turmeric
- ✓ One cinnamon stick
- ✓ ½ teaspoon salt
- ✓ 800g lamb neck fillet, cut into 2cm chunks
- ✓ 500g butternut squash, chopped into 1cm cubes
- ✓ 400g tin chopped tomatoes, plus half a can of water
- ✓ Two tablespoons fresh coriander (plus extra for garnish)
- ✓ 400g tin chickpeas, drained
- ✓ Buckwheat, couscous, flatbreads or rice to serve

Instructions:

- ✓ Preheat to 140C for your oven
- ✓ Drizzle in a large ovenproof casserole or cast casserole dish around two cubic cubes of olive oil. Slice onion and heat until the onions are

smooth but not browned, with a cover on for about 5 minutes.

- ✓ Ginger, chili, cumin, cinnamon, and turmeric are added to the grilled garlic. Cover well and cook with the lid for another 1 minute. If it gets too dry, add a sprinkle of water.
- ✓ Add next chunks of lamb. Add the butter, minced dates and tomato and a further half a can of water (100-200mL) to cover the meat in the onions and Spices. Mix well.
- ✓ Bring the tagine to a simmer, then place on the cover and place 1 hour and 15 minutes in your pre-heated oven.
- ✓ Add chopped butternut squash and drained chickpeas thirty minutes prior to the end of the cooking period. Put the cover on and back in the oven for the remaining 30 minutes of the preparation, bringing it together.
- ✓ Turn off the oven and mix with chopped coriander when tagine is finished. Serve with couscous, basmati or buckwheat.

Makes:4 servings Prep Time: 15 Mins Cook Time: 1 hour 15 Mins Total Time:1hour 30 Mins Calorie: 401kcal

Notes

If you don't own an ovenproof casserole or iron cast casserole dish, just bake the tagine in an ordinary bowl until it's in the oven and transfer it to an ordinary saucer before putting the tagine in the oven. Add an additional five minutes to cook to give more room to heat in the saucepan.

44. Grape And Melon Juice-Sirtfood Recipes

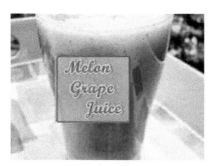

Ingredients:

- ✓ 1/2 cucumber, peel if necessary, halving, scraping seeds and roughing.
- ✓ 30 g youthful spinach leaves, removed stalks.

- ✓ 100 g red grapes without seeds
- ✓ 100 g of melon, washed, wished and cut cantaloupe.

Instruction:

- ✓ 1 In a juicer or blender, mix together until smooth.

Makes:1 servings Prep Time: 5 Mins Cook Time: 0 Mins Total Time:0 Mins Calorie: 125kcal

45. Chargrilled Beef With A Red Wine Jus, Onion Rings, Garlic Kale And Herb Roasted Potatoes-Sirtfood Recipes

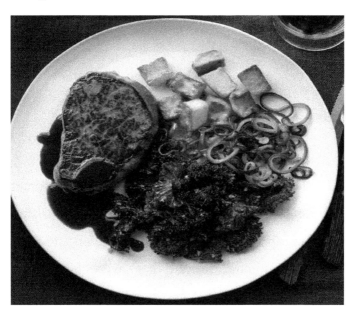

Ingredients:

- ✓ One tablespoon extra virgin olive oil
- ✓ 100g potatoes, peeled and cut into 2cm dice
- ✓ 50g red onion, sliced into rings
- ✓ 5g parsley, finely chopped
- ✓ One garlic clove, finely chopped
- ✓ 50g kale, sliced
- ✓ 40ml red wine
- ✓ 120–150g x 3.5cm-thick beef fillet steak or 2cm-thick sirloin steak
- ✓ 1 tsp tomato purée
- ✓ 150ml beef stock
- ✓ 1 tsp cornflour, dissolved in 1 tbsp water

Instructions:

- ✓ Oven power to 220 ° C / gas 7.
- ✓ Place the potatoes in a boiling pot and then drain for 4–5 minutes and put back to boil. In a roasting pan, apply one tablespoon of olive oil and roast 35-45 minutes in the hot oven. Placed the potatoes in order to ensure an even cooking per

10 minutes. Sprinkle the chopped Persil and mix well when cooked from the oven.

- ✓ Fry onion for 5 to 7 minutes in one teaspoon of oil until soft and beautifully caramelized over medium heat. Keep dry.
- ✓ Keeping it warm. Steam the kale and drain for about 2-3 minutes. Cook the goat softly, but not colored, in 1/2 teaspoon of oil for 1 minute. Attach the kale and brown before tender for another 1–2 minutes. Live wet. Remain dry.
- ✓ Heat a high-heat oven-proof frying pan to smoke. Cook the meat in 1⁄2 teaspoon of oil and mix in the heated bowl over medium-high flame, if you prefer your beef. If you want to use the beef mild, stitch the meat and move the bowl to a 220oC / gas seven furnace, such that the cooking may be done for the specified periods.
- ✓ Take the meat out of the pot and put it aside. To collect any residue of meat, add wine to the hot pot. Bubble with a balanced taste to slash the wine by half.

- ✓ Attach the pan to the stroked bowl, the tomato puree and the cornflour paste and thicken the sauce until you have the perfect consistency.
- ✓ Makes:2 servings Prep Time: 25 Mins Cook Time: 1 Hour 10 Mins Total Time:0 Mins Calorie: 425kcal

46. Kale And Blackcurrant Smoothie-Sirtfood Recipes

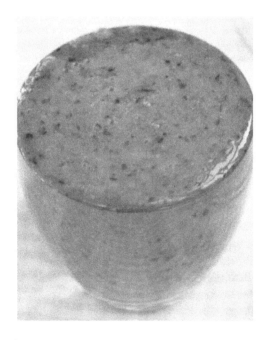

Ingredients:

- ✓ One cup freshly made green tea
- ✓ 2 tsp honey
- ✓ One ripe banana
- ✓ Ten baby kale leaves stalk removed
- ✓ Six ice cubes
- ✓ 40 g blackcurrants, washed and stalks removed

Instructions:

- ✓ Extract the honey until it is absorbed in the dry, green tea. Whisp in a mixer and add all ingredients into a fast processor. Serve right now.
- ✓ Makes:1 servings Prep Time: 0 Mins Cook Time: 3 Mins Total Time:0 Mins Calorie: 86kcal
- ✓

47. Buckwheat Pasta Salad-Sirtfood Recipes

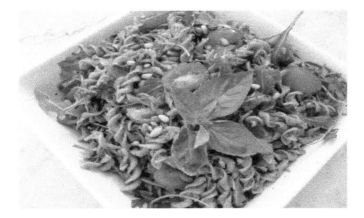

Instructions:

- ✓ large handful of rocket
- ✓ 50g buckwheat pasta(cooked according to the packet instructions)Sirtfood recipes
- ✓ Eight cherry tomatoes halved
- ✓ A small handful of basil leaves
- ✓ Ten olives
- ✓ 1/2 avocado, diced
- ✓ 20g pine nuts
- ✓ 1 tbsp extra virgin olive oil

Instructions:

- ✓ Mix all ingredients gently with the exception of the pine nut, and then arrange them on a plate or in a bowl.

Makes:1 servings Prep Time: 5 Mins Cook Time: 15 Mins Total Time:20 Mins Calorie: 195kcal

48. Greek Salad Skewers

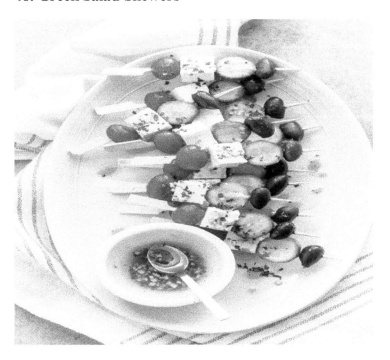

Ingredients:

- ✓ Eight large black olives
- ✓ Two wooden skewers, soaked in water for 30 minutes before use
- ✓ One yellow pepper, cut into eight squares
- ✓ Eight cherry tomatoes
- ✓ 100g (about 10cm) cucumber, cut into four slices and halved

- ✓ ½ red onion, cut in half and separated into eight pieces
- ✓ 100g feta, cut into eight cubes

For the dressing:

- ✓ Juice of ½ lemon
- ✓ 1 tbsp extra virgin olive oil
- ✓ ½ clove garlic, peeled and crushed
- ✓ 1 tsp balsamic vinegar
- ✓ Few oregano seeds, thinly sliced.
- ✓ Few basil leaves, thinly caught (or 1/2 tsp of drying, oregano and basil).
- ✓ Salt and black pepper seasoning.

Instructions:

- ✓ Thread per skewer in order with the ingredients in the salad: olive, tomato, red onion, cucumber, cucumber, basil, garlic, red onion, pepper, feta. Thinning the skewer in the order with the salad ingredients
- ✓ In a small pot, put all the dressing components and combine them thoroughly together. Verse the skewers around.

Makes:2 servings Prep Time: 5 Mins Cook Time: 5 Mins Total Time:10 Mins Calorie: 306kcal

49. Kale, Edamame And Tofu Curry-Sirtfood Recipes Sirtfood Recipes

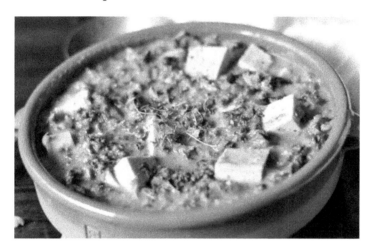

Warm curry and winter curry. Simple to hold cooled or frozen for another day.

Ingredients:

- ✓ A big onion, cut.
- ✓ One tbsp of rapeseed oil
- ✓ A big, fresh, peeled and grated thumb (7 cm).
- ✓ Four garlic cloves, peeled and rubbing.
- ✓ Taste for 1/2 tsp of turmeric on the ground.

- ✓ A red chili that is wanted and slimly cut.1 tsp paprika
- ✓ 1/4 tsp cayenne pepper
- ✓ 1 tsp salt
- ✓ 1/2 tsp ground cumin
- ✓ One liter boiling water
- ✓ 250g dried red lentils
- ✓ 200g firm tofu, chopped into cubes
- ✓ 50g frozen soya edamame beans
- ✓ Juice of 1 lime
- ✓ Two tomatoes, roughly chopped
- ✓ 200g kale leaves stalk removed and torn

Instructions

- ✓ Placed the oil in a heavy-bottom pan over the low-medium sun
- ✓ Attach the onion and cook for 5 minutes before inserting the garlic, ginger and chili, and cook for another 2 minutes.
- ✓ Remove the chili, cayenne, paprika, cumin and oil. Swirl once before inserting the red lentils and swirl again.

- ✓ Pour in boiling water and simmer for 10 minutes, then rising the heat and cook for another 20-30 minutes before the curry has a deep 'porridge' consistency.
- ✓ Add the rice, tofu and tomatoes and simmer for another 5 minutes. Add the lime juice and the kale leaves, then cook until the kale is soft.

Makes:4 servings Prep Time: 10 Mins Cook Time: 35 Mins Total Time:45 Mins Calorie: 342kcal

50. Chocolate Cupcakes With Matcha Icing-Sirtfood Recipes

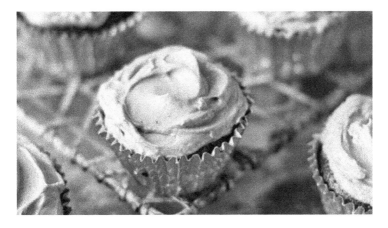

Ingredients:

- ✓ 200 g of caster sugar.
- ✓ 150 g flour self-raising.
- ✓ Salt with 1⁄2 tsp.
- ✓ Cocoa 60 g.
- ✓ Dairy 120ml.
- ✓ Fine espresso coffee with 1⁄2 tsp, decaf if preferred
- ✓ 50ml vegetable oil
- ✓ ½ tsp vanilla extract
- ✓ 120ml boiling water
- ✓ One egg

For the icing:

- ✓ 50g icing sugar
- ✓ 50g butter, at room temperature
- ✓ ½ tsp vanilla bean paste
- ✓ 1 tbsp matcha green tea powder
- ✓ 50g soft cream cheese

Instructions:

- ✓ Preheat the oven to a fan of 180C/160C, cover a cupcake tray with a paper or silicone cake shell.

- ✓ Place the rice, sugar, chocolate, salt and espresso powder in a large bowl and blend thoroughly.
- ✓ Apply the cream, vanilla extract, vegetable oil and egg to the dry ingredients and use an electric mixer until well mixed. Carefully dump gradually in the boiling water and pump at low speed before fully mixed.
- ✓ Using high speed to beat for another minute and attach fuel to the pump. The dough is even more oily than the normal cake blend. Have faith; it's going to taste amazing!
- ✓ Popular the batter equally between the cake cases. Each case of a cake will not be more than 3/4 whole. Bake in the oven for 15-18 minutes before the mixture has been tapped out. Remove from the oven and allow it to cool completely before icing.
- ✓ Mix the butter and icing sugar together until it is light and creamy. Add the matcha powder and vanilla, stir again. Attach the cream cheese and beat until smooth. Pipe or spray it over the cakes.

Makes:8 servings Prep Time: 10 Mins Cook Time: 30 Mins
Total Time:40 Mins Calorie: 234kcal

Conclusion

The Sirtfood Diet, created by nutritionists Aidan Goggins
and Glen Matten, is the latest nutrition pattern to sweep the
world, and the creators claim that it works to activate the
"lean gene" of your body. The diet is a two-part approach
and focuses on consuming foods rich in sirtuin, as well as
calorie restriction.

Sirtuins are a group of seven proteins that protect our cells
in the body from dying or being inflamed due to disease,
explains nutritionist Michele, adding that research has also
found that proteins can help regulate your metabolism,
increase muscle and burn. Vet. polyphenols, Michele says,
are micronutrients packed with antioxidants that have been
found to improve digestion and neurodegenerative and
cardiovascular diseases.

To begin dieting, participants should follow a two-week
plan, which includes the reduction of calorie consumption
and the consumption of "green sirt food" juices."During the

first week, you will limit [calorie] intake to 1,000 calories, which includes consuming three sirtfood-green juices and one meal rich in sirtfood per day," Michele shares. "The next week, she raises her intake to 1,500 calories a day and eats two food-rich meals and two green juices."

In the long run, no specific diet exists, but a high-nutritional diet plan is recommended, along with incorporating the green juices that are characteristic of the diet. The creators of the diet claim that the diet will lead to rapid weight loss while retaining muscle and mass and protecting you from chronic illnesses.